Diary Of A
Bipolar Survivor

You can't control the waves but you can always learn to surf.

[signature]

Elaine Fogarty

chipmunkapublishing
the mental health publisher

Elaine Fogarty

Published by
Chipmunkapublishing
PO Box 6872
Brentwood
Essex CM13 1ZT
United Kingdom

http://www.chipmunkapublishing.com

Edited by Fran Harvey

ISBN   978-1-84991-974-6

Chipmunkapublishing gratefully acknowledge the support of Arts Council England.

For Colin & Dean.
Because I have been blessed with two soul mates.

With thanks to
My family, for their unconditional love and support
all these years.

There's a book by A.A. Milne,
About a little bear.
You really ought to read it;
There's lots of wisdom there.
Of course it makes young children smile,
But there's a lesson for adults too.
Don't worry about what could happen;
Your fears may not come true.

(Elaine Fogarty)

Author Biography

At the young age of just 13, Elaine was struggling with dark thoughts and wrote the poem 'suicide'; her poetry and scribbled journal notes were a valued means of expression and exploration. In following years she started to self harm and in her twenties she began to receive periodic treatment for depression. Elaine found herself in suicidal crisis three times, but survived each by the grace of a stranger. In 2006 she found herself back in that darkest of places and decided to make a stand; she gathered her journal notes and sat nervously with her GP. After four weeks on a psychiatric ward, the demon was finally named: bipolar II.

Elaine now acknowledges her bipolar disorder, anxiety issues, self harm and OCD. Thirty years on, she denies them strength born of secrecy and chooses instead to be totally open about her mental illness.

Elaine was born in 1967 in Portadown, Northern Ireland. She has been with her husband Colin for over 28 years, and still lives in her hometown with him and B'Elanna the tailless cat. She spent many years moving from job to job, but is now happily settled in an administrative post with a local wholesale business. Elaine enjoys film and theatre, good food shared with good friends, and the sense of connection afforded her by social networking online.

Elaine Fogarty

Preface

Daisies are quite my favourite flower. They are so cheery and always make me smile. I identify with them because they, too, live their lives facing stigma. The humble daisy is beautiful and intricate in design, but only children and a small handful of adults see that beauty; others choose to ignore its merits and label it a 'weed'. We all know how damaging labels can be, doubly so when used in ignorance. The poor daisy is driven from our lawns and verges as if it carried some virulent disease. Lawns are un-accepting of anything that is not green: this is discrimination – this is stigma – this is, unfortunately, the way of our world. The daisy and I are kindred spirits and I aspire to its survival skills. As you can see in the cover picture, a lone daisy will find purchase in seemingly inhospitable ground; it will tenaciously grow despite the challenges of weather and footfall. The daisy has faith in its own ability and invests all its energy in life; it never gives up, never. Seasons come and go for my little friend just as they do for me, but the daisy continues to look to the sun for support, tracking it as it moves across the sky.

I have learnt so much from my friend the daisy. Until recent years, I went to great lengths to hide my problems. I was in denial; I didn't want to accept the label of mental illness. No one knew the full extent of my struggle and, with the exception of Samaritan helpline volunteers, no one ever knew that I'd come close to killing myself more than once. My scribbled poetry and journal notes kept me safe by allowing me to vent; to articulate the frightening, jumbled mess of emotions inside me. I never intended to share these notes, but more than thirty years on, I finally feel able to allow others into my secret world. My old English teacher would tell you that I was not particularly skilled, couldn't spell to save my life and was way too fond of commas – but still, I wrote. Here you will read raw diary entries; I haven't 'prettied' the text up or made unnecessary changes. These pages should give you some measure of insight into a bipolar mind. I am the one in four; I have a mental illness.

It is what it is – no more.

Elaine Fogarty

Table of contents

Elaine Fogarty

Poetry selection

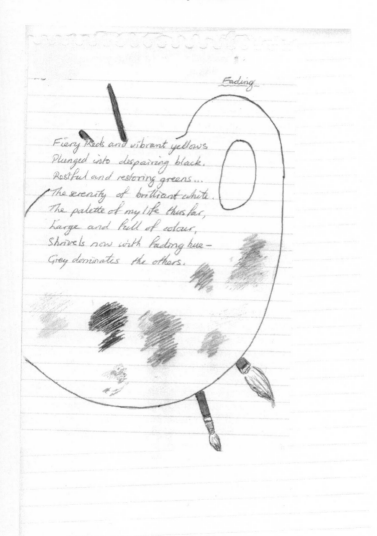

Fading

Fiery Reds and vibrant yellows
Plunged into despairing black.
Restful and restoring greens...
The serenity of brilliant white.
The palette of my life thus far,
Large and full of colour,
Shrivels now with fading hue –
Grey dominates the others.

The natural world

Silent combat

The sky used to flow like a river,
White ripples on soft blue,
Now it's forced ever upwards,
Almost out of view.
Clouds push for space among the rooftops,
Bricks stand proudly in their ranks.
The grass and flowers are in subjection,
But a few rebels still fight back.
The invader's strength is growing;
The battle almost won,
In this, the slow and silent war,
That kills without a gun.

Evening shower

Ringlets of water spread and fade
As the rain falls gently down,
And as I watch I fill with awe
At the beauty that's around.
Crystals of moisture hang from leaves,
Priceless gems on spider's webs;
God's own rainbow by the roadside,
But still the world walks by.

How like man it is indeed
To ignore such simple beauty.
God's world becomes man's world,
And all is self and envy.
What of a newborn babe?
A mother's smile?
Two lovers in the rain?
Friendship and forgiveness?
No, still the world walks by.

People of the rain

Rain makes philosophers of us all.
Thoughts dance with ease to its tune
And tears have no enemy.
It embraces the anxious and the lonely
As they share their secret pain.
It befriends the loving couple
As they plan their lives together.
Their thoughts flow with the droplets of water
And saturate the air;
They rise, and blend, and fall again
As someone else's inspiration.

Playful nature

Jostling playfully for space,
Reaching out towards the sun,
Waving and blowing kisses to all who pass,
Flowers encourage a sense of fun.
Undeterred by cold indifference
Each shares its radiant smile,
Engaging in happy conversation
With all who pause a while.

Regeneration

A pervading scent of renewal hangs delicately in the air.
Nothing is impossible now,
In this world reborn of rain.
From behind the veil of indifference emerges a living Earth.
All illusion is gone now,
In this world reborn of rain.

Encounter

Roadside red poppies
Dancing gaily in the wind.
A joyous splash of vivid colour
Too soon passed.
And yet I wonder...
What life they have?
What they see?
And why they choose to speak to me?

The Promise

With a gentle kiss, this morning
The sun woke me from my sleep
And, returning yet another day,
Said, "This promise I will keep:
To softly invite each child to wake
And shed warm light upon their day;
To trace the sky and count the hours,
And help them on their way.
To share my light and warmth with all,
Regardless of colour or creed;
To bring life to nature's garden
So all can happily feed.
To be a friend and constant reminder
Of the good that's in this world;
To uplift, inspire and encourage
'Til night's canvas is unfurled."

Emotions

Building

All my life I've been building walls
Between my friends and me:
With each brick I laid up hope
of my security.
What couldn't touch me couldn't hurt,
of this I had no doubt.
That's why I built my walls so high
And kept the world out.
But I got lonely trapped inside
My little self-made cell,
For in keeping out the hurtin'
I kept lovin' out as well.
Now I really want to free myself
But I'm just too scared to try;
And no one else may enter,
For I built my walls too high.

Missing you

I awoke with a smile and turned over,
Reaching out to hold you.
I could feel your warm body nestled beside me,
I could hear you breathe slow and calm;
But my arm fell heavy without you
And suddenly I was alone.
I gathered the covers up round me,
Pulling them close to my face.
Safe in their comfort I closed my eyes,
Drifting slowly back into the dream:
The dream that would one day be real.

Escape

Show me a window and open it wide,
Or even a little,
But let in some light.

Where has the sky gone?
Why is it so dark?
Oh, close it again and at least leave me hope.

Let me imagine a clear blue sky,
With soft white clouds and birds soaring high.
Let me imagine the life they have;
Let me imagine the freedom they have.
If there's no hope for my life,
Let me live theirs.

The wall

Just this once I let down my guard
And the wall began to crack;
Just this once I peered through the hole,
And saw the world wasn't just black and white.
Dare I knock out a brick to see further?
Dare I reach for the other side?
Or stay here within my fortress,
And quietly, safely, hide?
Hidden safe behind my walls,
What couldn't touch me couldn't hurt.
So should I bravely reach for sky?
Or sit here in the dirt?
I've wasted my life building walls,
Too scared to really live.
So now I've got to take a risk
And see what the world has to give.

Love

Love should join a union;
It's overworked and underpaid.
The word is given no respect,
Especially in bed.
It's got such a reputation,
It may just go on strike.
Then what would we say,
When we mean much more than Like?

A quiver of hearts

Cupid's little arrow
Has grown into a long, piercing blade.
It twists and tears at my heart...
But love -
Love is in the pain.
But love -
Love is in the healing.
But love -
Love is a survivor.

Clouds

Some dark thoughts like clouds drift by,
Barely acknowledged,
While others, heavy with rain,
Pause to make themselves better heard.
Clouds pass.
The warm sun re-asserts itself
And hangs for a time
In a sky pregnant with promise -
The clouds will come again.

When clear blue skies present themselves
I view them with suspicion;
I have grown accustomed to the clouds
And a part of me aches in their absence.

The first time in ages

Is happiness just a better-than-yesterday feeling?
Or is it something much more profound?
Is it love?
Is it friendship?
Or just contentment?
Whatever it is,
It's been found.
I'm finding it hard to recognise
And even harder to define.
I just know, for the first time in ages,
Happiness
Is finally mine.

Echoes

The view through the window is boring,
Like a dusty picture hanging on the wall.
But I stare at it anyway,
Daydreaming.
If I turn my head, I'll face you,
And I'd rather daydream in secret
Than be seen to watch you;
Than to see you watch me.
I can feel your eyes moving across me.
I can hear your thoughts echo mine.
I can almost feel your touch
And that scares me.
It feels too good to be a memory,
Yet too good to be real.

The future revisited

Under cover of darkness,
It comes to me.
Again
And again:
The dream that cries out to live.

Daylight darkness

Another day:
Another nightmare of confusion.
Decisions, problems, hopes and fears
Emerge from their lairs and wait.
Security is a thing of the past.
Each step I take leads me
Further into the light of day and
Further into the darkness of anxiety.
I can sense them lurking there -
Behind me, watching, waiting.

Why suicide?

Now I'm finally gone, will you sob and cry?
Will you silently ponder the reason why
I should have chosen this way to die?

I couldn't find a way to fully explain or tame
The crippling, crushing, relentless pain.
It's not your fault – I am to blame.

I should have shouted until I was heard.
I should have fought longer, harder, found the words
To make real the unthinkable and absurd.

I wanted to live, but finally chose to die,
To escape, and spare others my contagious pain.
As for that final straw? Even I can't answer why.

Waiting

I miss the sound of your voice,
The touch of your hand,
And the warmth of your breath on my skin.
I miss holding you tight
And you must know I dream
Of having you near me again.
I want you,
I need you,
And, though you're not with me,
My thoughts still echo your name.

Elaine Fogarty

The question

Why? – I wish I could tell you.
I really do.
I wish I could go back in time
And make you understand how it felt.
Why did I kill myself?
Because I was trapped in a glass cell
And death offered up a key.
Because I felt so alone and desperate
And no one wanted to hear me scream.
It made them uncomfortable;
It frightened them.
My bloodied hands beat against the glass
But it would not break.
Exhausted and still in pain,
I had to escape.
Had there been another way
I would have taken it.

Pen of tears

I'd like to cry, but it won't come out.
I need to cry – to get it all out.
I'd like to talk, but I can't explain.
I need to talk – to ease the pain.
So instead, I write
To let feelings loose,
But no one ever reads it –
So then – what's the use?
I write,
And then I listen,
To the problems of my friends;
Push my own down even deeper,
And go on to pretend.

Together

Last night you held me in your arms
And we made love beneath the stars.
Every inch of my body was alive to your touch;
There seemed no other movement but ours.
The night was calm and beautifully still,
But for a welcome, gentle breeze.
In my ear, your loving whispers
Spoke of a thousand ways to please.
My hands ran softly through your hair,
And drew you near to steal a kiss;
Passion growing ever stronger now,
Fuelled by just a hint of risk.
Your face, bathed in moonlight,
Carried its usual playful smile.
I gazed deeply into your shining eyes
And lingered just a while.
The hands of time were running slow;
Minutes together felt like hours.
Nothing else in the world could matter;
This time was entirely ours.
Drawn instinctively together,
Our bodies intertwined.
More than love, more than lust,
The feeling couldn't be defined.
It was more the perfect meeting
Of two equally needy souls;
Two people meant to be together,
But playing different roles.
Life conspired to part us,
At least that's the way it seemed,
But at last we were together –

Together in my dreams.

Elaine Fogarty

The hunt

Guilt, like many carnivores,
Hunts in the broad light of day.
Quiet and unnoticed,
It sleeps through the night,
Arising with the sun to prey.
Carefully stalking,
With a hunger unending,
It hunts upon the stray.

Fading

Fiery reds and vibrant yellows
Plunged into despairing black.
Restful and restoring greens…
The serenity of brilliant white.
The palette of my life, thus far
Large and full of colour,
Shrivels now with fading hue –
Grey dominates the others.

The return

Weariness washes over me
And drips from every pore.
Eyes close into the darkness
And I'm heavy to the core.
Time slows and spins about me.
I've been here before.

Wishes

Anxiety enveloping me, depression stalking me
And the stench of loneliness hangs heavy in the air.
Waves of nausea and panic carry me through the day
till I come to rest,
Trapped in the very corner of hopelessness,
Tasting the saltiness of uncontrollable tears.
Depression lurks in the shadows and whispers to me, telling tales
of things to come,
And that scares me.
I wish it all to go away and, were my wishes like drops of rain,
They still could not nourish the seed of hope.

Foundations

Our relationship is like a home,
It should keep us safe and dry.
But lately I've been noticing
That safety is a lie.
Maintenance has been neglected
Upkeep has been so poor.
Foundations are slowly sinking
And there's damp all round the door.
Was I really then the only one
To see the warning signs?
I told you oh so many times
But you think that all is fine.
The house that I so rely on
Is crumbling round my head.
I'm so desperate and alone
Said all I could have said.
I can't make you see it
How I wish that you could know
How very much I need you
And how I love you so.

The angel's call

Words spoken with a smile, masquerading as a jest,
Cling to the very air she breathes and so infect and breed – infest.
They build upon past injuries and unintended harm.
They seethe, and writhe, and creep, and crawl,
'Til little else is left at all.
Still, a hollow shell bereft of hope,
That grieving love in darkness gropes,
Amid the thoughts to end it all,
And listens for the angel's call.

The rock

The same rock that I climb upon
To bask in summer sun
Remains a solid anchor
When winter storms freshly come.
Water that once playfully flowed
Around my shifting toes
Swells and rages about me,
Attacking as it goes.
But to that Rock I tightly cling,
On its tested strength rely,
These waters shall not claim me –
Today I shall not die.

Another time, another place

Last night
I blamed the storm
For keeping me awake.
This morning
The storm is gone,
And I'm left with the truth.
You crept into my thoughts
And linger still.
This morning
There are no regrets;
Just the fear of hope.

Burning as it rose

I wasn't afraid at the time,
But then fear rose like bile
And burnt me from inside.
Lingering yet a while,
It burrowed deep inside me,
Steeled by hateful guile,
There took root and quickly grew,
Notch by notch, it turned the dial.

On the edge of forever

There's a cliff on the edge of forever,
I know because I walk by
To drink in the air,
To admire the view
And let the time pass by.

Often I look down and think,
To step on off that cliff,
To fall at long last,
Into nothingness,
To all, my parting gift.

I can sit with my legs dangling,
Alone with all my pain,
Wishing to fall,
Wanting to fall,
Then change my mind again.

There's a cliff on the edge of forever.
It scares me to know it well,
Needing it so badly,
Fearing it so badly,
None believe so, then, why tell?

Shameful jealousy

Words spoken softly with concern,
Drift across the quiet room;
Their intent and meaning understood,
Yet they invite a sense of gloom.
With their enquiry and concern
I whole-heartedly agree,
Yet I wonder – when I was suicidal,
Why they never came to me?

I too had really struggled,
I too knew crippling pain.
My self-esteem is crushed to learn,
A difference is quite plain.
Even though I chose to talk,
Dared to speak of suicide,
Words spoken softly with concern,
In this room did not abide.

My jealousy now my sorry shame,
I pondered recent times;
The polar difference sadly clear,
A sense of injury climbs.
It rises up from deep inside me.
It fills my every thought.
It seeps into my purest self.
Answers there are newly sought.

Social comment

Does he?

As a matter of fact, I don't take sugar.
Thank you all the same.

Why, Mrs Jones, you've gone so pale.
Was it something that I said?
Why so surprised to hear me speak?
Would you rather I drooled instead?
I'm sorry to be so sarcastic,
But you're driving me insane.
Just because I'm in a wheel chair
Doesn't mean I've lost my brain.

A question of advertising

Which came first -
The chart hit or the advert?
The satisfied customer
Or the hard sell?
They're all newly improved now,
With at least 10% free.
They're travel size and family size,
With a money-back guarantee.
They've got bright designer packets
Endorsed by famous names;
They're all cheaper than their rivals,
But all seem to be the same.

Which came first -
The chart hit or the advert?
It doesn't matter what they are,
They'll always try to sell.

Elaine Fogarty

Bus shelter

Among the crushed beer cans
And the empty cigarette packets
Lay a crumpled carrier bag.
It was hardly worth noticing,
Except that it wasn't empty.
It kicked
And it struggled
To survive its first day.

That was the problem;
He had always been considered
IT.
He only survived this long
Because money doesn't grow on trees,
And surgeons have to be paid.

The colour of money

Money -
The be all and end all,
The god of our time.
Mother of greed.
Father of crime.
Its lure is strong,
Its promise is grand.
Money is power.
The powerful stand.
Money can buy diamonds,
Missiles and guns.
Money could buy food;
Work could be done.
Millions still lie dying.
The world just doesn't see.
Money clouds our vision;
Money is all we see.

Charity

Yet another envelope through the door,
Yet another rattling box on the street,
Yet another television appeal.
Yet another chance to give life and hope.
Yet another turns away.
Yet another dies today.

The list

Two of these: they're ozone friendly.
Some of this recycled stuff.
Four of these: they're high in fibre.
Clingfilm safe enough.
Some packets, no E numbers.
Eggs, if I really must.
Two more tubs of low fat
And a tin without some rust.
Three of these: lower calories,
And fresh anything green.
Pay it all with plastic
And drive on home lead-free.

Evening viewing

Good evening. Here is the news:

There's been another strike;
They're fighting for more pay.
There's been another murder;
The second one today.
There's been another meeting;
To bargain for world peace.
There's been another jailing;
He raped his own niece.
There's been another closure;
The investors won't be paid.
There's been another air crash;
Two hundred people dead.
There'll be another news show
On tomorrow night,
But will the news be old news?
We suspect it might.

Denim culture

People just aren't the same any more.
They wear t-shirts,
Like badges to announce who they are.
There's a whole new denim culture now,
With cotton identity cards.
Everyone feels they have to belong.
The sheep queue up to be rebels
And buy the latest offensive design.
The people in suits get even richer,
Laughing as the cash keeps rolling in.
They know they're not just selling t-shirts;
They're selling dreams.
Dreams will always sell.

A change of season

Perhaps we should have Christmas
At a different time of year,
When the music is quieter,
The lights are dimmer
And there's less of the Christmas cheer.
When the tills are quieter,
The parties fewer
And people have time to hear.

Extinct is forever

Extinct is forever.
Forever could start today.
Thousands of different species
Are quietly slipping away.
Soon there'll be only pictures,
Video tape and slides.
Soon there'll be only memories
Of the creatures who have died.
Soon we've got to save them;
Someone has to try.
Soon we have to make a stand,
Before the chance has passed us by.

Voice of the condemned

I'm all alone, hopelessly condemned for something
I had no control over. When I need all your
Love and compassion you desert me,
And yet regard yourself as a warm,
Understanding person, morally secure.
You know nothing, and your ignorance is surpassed
Only by your conceit. Your cruel conceit.
By your decision, I came into being;
Yet you reject me as nothing more than
A nameless consequence of a mistake.
You speak of your right as a woman,
To do as you please with your own body -
That pitiful shell that houses a soul, forever
Blackened with hypocrisy and conceit.
You refuse to acknowledge my rights.
My right to live, to see for myself the
Chaos of society, the violence, the hatred
Caused by you and others like you:
My right to see too, the hidden beauty of the world,
To search out for myself that love carried
Deep within each person, often hidden through shame.
Having created life, are you too selfish to
Allow it to continue? To you, I'm just an
Inconvenience, but I refuse to die to make your
Life more comfortable, and then to be forgotten.
If you deny me the fundamental right to life
My tiny body may cease to exist, but I will
Live on in your memory.
I refuse to be rejected and forgotten!
Your decision; your mistake; your guilt.

Just one man

Don't blame me for global warming
Or the rising of the seas.
Don't blame me for loss of species,
Precious plants or ancient trees.
I only take what's due to me,
My family still needs fed.
You have no right to stop me.
Go save the whales instead!

The price of Christmas

Everyone finds themselves humming
To Christmas tunes they hate:
An endless barrage of Christmas cheer
Assaults each and every ear.
Bright lights, holly and tinsel,
Christmas cards and Christmas gifts.
What to choose? How to decide?
Everyone's under pressure to buy.

Learning

Children cannot survive in today's twisted society;
From the moment they're born they're under threat.
We feed them a poison which erodes the moral fibre.
Before they reach the age of six they're mature;
They've learnt to lie, to cheat, to live for self alone.
We destroy the honesty they were born with,
And with it destroy our hope of survival.
Once, society meant caring, co-operation and trust,
But we live by dishonesty and selfishness.
Now society is crumbling,
Folding in on itself and dying:
The only ones who can save it are the children -
If we'll let them.

Dedicated pieces

Closed

A tiny unlabelled bottle hides under layers of dust,
Pushed right to the back of the pharmacy shelf.
Ignored or forgotten for years;
Never more needed than now.
All over the world, hundreds of men and women
Search for it; even more desperately need it.
The little bottle may never be discovered:
The whole building is scheduled for demolition.
By the end of the year it will be gone,
Gone forever.
The pharmacy will be closed.

(Dedicated to the men and women who try to protect our rainforests.)

Unspoken love

Unspoken love finds its expression
With the reassuring clasp of hands,
With the silence of a loving gaze,
With the tender touch of lips.
This love has a voice beyond words.

A love complete within this union,
Together at last, one beautiful whole.
This marriage uniting two wonderful people,
As it finally unites one beautiful soul.
A love secure and reassuring,
With hidden depths; much to explore,
This is a love to face life's challenge
And allow flightless dreams to soar.

(For Kara and Simon on their wedding day.)

42

The answer to life is 42
But the question was too vague.
So they took the form of mice and then,
For crumbs of cheese did beg.

They ran their mazes and kept low,
Observing all mankind.
The Earth itself commissioned,
The question urgently to find.

Ten million years went by.
The Vogons went and blew it up.
The mice were really most displeased,
For they'd paid pre-interrupt.

The ultimate question almost found,
A girl solved the many clues.
Then the organic matrix was destroyed,
But our hero Arthur was rescued.

His friend Ford turned out to be an alien,
And together they hitched a lift
Aboard an orbiting Vogon craft,
Until in space were set adrift.

They should have died, they really should.
But against all odds were saved.
A guy with two heads, an old girlfriend.
Arthur didn't know how to behave.

They joined Zaphod's bizarre quest,
Chasing down the vaguest of ideas.
And against all odds they finally found
The planet of Magerathea.

Its trade, building custom planets,
Long lost in legend, doubted to exist.
They'd been paid to built a computer,
And now the mice were pissed.

By the time Arthur saw the factory floor,
A total rebuild had begun.
Sadly though, they needed his brain
To make the system run.

It was bad enough to lose his home,
To find himself in space instead,
But he wasn't about to die today,
So squished the mice quite dead.

Dead mice meant no clients,
But Earth 2 was almost done.
They offered Arthur a place there,
But by now the girl he'd won.

Our story doesn't end here at all,
For with an improbability drive,
Arthur and Trillian had more options
Than anyone alive.

Of course there are more details,
A crazy rollercoaster ride…
If curious what else happened
Then just ask The Guide.

(For Douglas Adams, author of 'The Hitchhiker's Guide to the Galaxy – A trilogy in five parts'. Thank you for the one book that can always make me smile.)

Blessing

In this world of uncertainty, may you always be guided by the certainty of your love.

May you be friends, as well as lovers.
May you feel comfort in silence shared.
May you welcome tears, as well as laughter.
May your inner voices be always heard.
May you know the joy of playful days.
May you happily work side by side.
May you always see each other as you are today –
Forever a Groom and his Bride.

(For Catherine and David on their wedding day.)

Hugs

In a place beyond space and time,
Words do not exist.
Safe within a heartfelt hug,
Expression is sublime.

Emotion saturates the air,
Arms entwine so tight.
A free exchange of smiles and tears,
Eternity to share.

(For Dean, a true friend.)

When I die

Don't dwell long in loss and sadness.
Don't leave your eyes in tear.
Don't worry about the future
Because, my love,
I'm here.
Feel my hand in the breeze that brushes your cheek.
Feel my kiss in the warmth of the sun.
Feel my love in every breath drawn in.
I cannot leave you.
We are one.

(For my husband Colin.)

Lost in the moment

I'm happy when I'm in your arms,
As if caught in some fleeting vacuum.
A happiness otherwise elusive,
At least is real then, tangible and intense.
Nothing in the world can touch,
Let alone, hurt me.
I am completely and utterly lost.
Lost in the moment.
Lost in my dreams.

(For my husband, Colin.)

Ode to Aunty

We were standin' in the post office
In that stupid zigzag queue,
Waiting in vain for the line to move
And chatting – as you do.

Well, we complained about the weather,
And slegged off more than one,
But the queue wasn't for movin'
Our wait had just begun.

Says I: "You'll never guess who's 50!"
Says she: "Go on, then, who?"
Says I: "It's only Irene Loney."
Says she: "What? Irene who?"

"Auch," says I. "You're bound to remember
Ellen Lucinda Irene.
She went to school in Milltown,
Mind? She hated Gertie Magee."

Says she: "Then was there a sister Mary?"
"That's it," says I. "You're right."
"Ay," says she, "indeed I am.
Do you know if they still fight?"

Says I: "Yeah, even with eight years difference,
They surely used to fight.
They were at it once when the minister called,
I'm sure that was a sight."

"So what's she doin' these days?" says she,
"Did she marry? Settle down?
What about ol' Bertie from Ballymena,
Or even Tommy? You know, from town?"

"No," says I. "She never did,
She's an unclaimed treasure for sure.
Mind you, if she had a married,
He might a headed for the door.

He couldn't have kept up wi' her,
Traipsin' round all those car boot sales;
She always has to go home with a bargain,
And generally – she never fails."

Says she: "Ay, do ye know I think I saw her
A while back, at Chambers Park,
Carrying a stupid lookin' trolley thing,
That must have been out of the ark!

So do ye be round to see her often?
Suppose her house is always full?"
"Indeed," says I, "Ye must be joking
She hates a house that's full!"

She hates those after-concert suppers,
Where the visitors just won't go;
They sit there 'til all hours chattin'
And the endless gossip flows.

An' all the time, she's dreamin'
Of a peaceful swig o' tay,
Wishin' they'd all just disappear,
--Give her head a holiday."

Say I: "And do you remember
That little grey mini she drove?
You mind, she rammed it into Richie's pig house,
Off the Dungannon Road.

Still she didn't crash the brown fiesta,
Drove it 13 year!
Drove it really carefully,
I mean she never found 3rd gear!

Once she was on the motorway
Doin' 20, if ye please!
No lights and no seat belt; it was 20 to 1
She sailed along with ease.

Sure, she saw the car behind her,
But gave it not a thought -
Until they stopped her 'n said she'd been drinkin',
Then she really got distraught.

"Oh no," says Irene "I've not been drinkin',
I've only had a couple of Shloer.
I've really just been dilly- dallying,
To breathalyse me wouldn't be fair.""

"That's a laugh," says she, "for sure.
So tell me, where's she workin' in?
I mind she used to work in Vance's,
Before the flour annoyed her skin."

"That's right," says I, "She left them,
And went to the Mayfair to work.
Always there before the world's awake,
  -- That's just her little quirk!"

By now, the queue was moving a little,
We were edging to the front,
I swear if it wasn't for me premium bonds,
I'd let them go an' bunt!

So we turned again to chattin',
And back to poor Irene,
Who is always moanin' and groanin', lamentin' and gruntin',
But never has happier been.

"Do ye know?" says I, "she's into antiques now,
Pink glass and the such I fear.
I'm sure she'll soon get sick of that,
When she realises it's so dear!

I can just picture her trapsin' roun' shops and stalls,
Lookin' for a bargain clear,
Then just an hour later sayin' to friends,
I'm browned off, get me out of here!"

Says I: "She'd be happier at home,
Tuckin' into a huge big fry.
She loves them, ye know, but they hate her,
No matter how she tries.

For a woman who loves her food,
It's a shame te trouble she's prone,
She can't eat scallions, tomatoes or turkey,
Without a dose of gravel stone!"

"Gravel stone? What's that?" says she.
"Ah," says I, "it's Gaviscon!"
The woman may be 50 now,
But she's still slow to catch on!

39

Indeed, she may well need it,
Come Sunday when she's ill.
By Monday, she'll be right as rain,
For she has her work to go till.

For it wouldn't do te miss it;
It wouldn't go down well,
She'd have a face just like a pismire,
As if the sky had fell.

Says she: "All this talk of Irene,
Has made me curious for sure,
I'll finish me shoppin', pay me bills,
And go knock on 'er door."

Then a voice boomed loud behind us,
"No need, she'll not be in.
Ye see she's been here all the while – just lis'nin'
And what a laugh it's been!"

(For Irene Loney)

Identity crisis

Thatched cottages and petrol bombs,
Leprechauns and guns,
Irish stew and murder,
Rolling hills and buried sons.
The rest of the world doesn't know us;
Most people don't even care,
But they'll continue to make their judgements,
Making sure opinions air.
It's up to us to put them straight;
To tell them who we are,
But until we actually find that out,
We won't get very far.

(Dedicated to the people of Northern Ireland with the hope of eventual peace.)

No

'Oh, I know what you mean.
That's totally normal.'
No.
No, it's not, and NO, you don't.

(For those who face indifference.)

Happy 10th birthday

They say life only begins at 40,
So I guess that makes you 10.
You'll rarely see a better chance
To act like a child again!
Now you've had a few years practice,
With all the laughter and tears,
Before wandering into First Trust Bank
And staying 30 years!
So all grown up, and three kids on,
With a husband by your side,
Now's not the time to be slowin' down.
Don't let a number make you hide!
Keep dancin' on a Monday night.
Get out there and have some fun.
Keep finding new ways to really enjoy
Florida's playground in the sun.

Make the most of these coming years.
By the same token you'll sure see
You're headin' now to puberty,
A cheeky teenager soon to be.
What a chance to shake things up,
Show others how it's done…
Get out there NOW Doretta –
The rebellious years have just begun!
Grow older quite disgracefully,
Do all you've ever wanted to.

Pay heed to no one's disapproval,
After all – what do children do?
Go to new places, make new friends,
Indulge in silliness – No Fear!
And start planning a major party,
To celebrate your 18th year!

(Dedicated to Doretta on the occasion of her 50th birthday celebration.)

Soul mates

An hour with you
Disperses the gloom
That clouds so many days.
A minute with you
Puts a smile on my face
And dissolves my problems away.
Talking to you
Leaves me feeling secure
And ready, come what may.
But best of all,
Knowing you
Has made me luckier than I can say.

(For Dean.)

And all of the rest

On the reading of poetry

If Milton or Shakespeare or Keats
Were responsible for writing this piece,
You would read it
And praise it -
See their genius in it,
Nod your head in an all-knowing way.
But because I wrote it down,
You read and you frown.
But just wait -
I'll be famous some day.

This moment

As I look into the eyes of this new day
I see the colour of peace and the light of love.
As I rest in the arms of this new day,
Hours embrace and minutes offer up the sweetest kiss.
As I walk hand in hand with this new day,
My breath echoes the music of creation.
All that exists, exists here.
All that is possible, is possible here.

Eternity pours into this moment.

On the shelf

They stand like an army on parade;
Making a statement
For anyone who comes near.
They'll never be read,
But they look good,
And that's what matters.
People judge me by their covers
And I like what they see.

Perhaps

Today is my birthday,
But I won't get up; I'll stay here in bed.
I couldn't go downstairs, not today.
Downstairs I can hear the laughter.
I can imagine them huddling together,
Excitedly tearing the paper off their presents
And smiling above their disappointment.
They'll go in to dinner soon
And eat all that fancy food,
Even though they're not hungry.
There won't be a place set for me.
There never is.
But it's my birthday!

What does that matter to them?
They've got their cards and their presents;
They're having a good time.
Perhaps next year they'll remember me.
Perhaps I'll get a card or a present or...
Perhaps they'll even come talk to me a while.
Perhaps.

Between the lines

Is poetry a window to the soul?

Look between the lines.

Can you see emotion swelling?
Can you feel it reaching out?
Can you hear the secret joys and pains
That long to rise and shout?
Can you see it?
Can you feel it?
Can you tell what the poem is about?

Browsing

The other day I stumbled upon a library.
I'd never really noticed it before,
But it seemed strangely inviting,
Luring me in to browse around.
Inside it was vaguely familiar,
A little old-fashioned at first, but
Warm and comforting.
As I moved from section to section
Curiosity gave way to surprising interest.
Like a child in a toy shop
I soon became bewildered by choice.
History, law, poetry, biography,
Published letters and real-life drama.
I flicked through stories of war,
Adultery and betrayal,
Political unrest and crime.
I saw poetry so beautiful it read like music,
And stories of lives that could have been mine.
And stories of love...
Now those were the best ones,
Scattered around to outnumber the rest.
One in particular caught my eye:
A heartrending tale of father and child.
As a ransom for loved ones
He sends his own son;
His life for theirs – a painful exchange.
I turned to the closing chapter
And emotion in me swelled.
It was all so painful, so beautiful,
So real,
Too real.
So I put the library back on the shelf.

Someone special

Anyone
Can write a poem:
It takes someone special
To let
A poem write itself.

Elaine Fogarty

Games

Time likes to play games.
It moves quickly when you want it most
And at a snail's pace when you don't.
Happy hours pass just as minutes,
Cascading by, out of control.
Painful moments creep by like the dead of night.

Time likes to play games:
Time knows it will always win.

A wedding gift

In the hope it's never opened,
This box was wrapped up tight.
Today, as you spoke your wedding vows,
We trapped them safe inside.

Keep it safely stowed away,
The words forever sealed.
With them kisses, smiles and laughter,
And all the love you feel.
If memories ever begin to fade,
If the world seems dull and grey,
Just take this out again and hold it,
To remind you of today.

Dial-a-dream

Sleep regrets he's not available at the moment -
But if you'd like to leave your problems,
Daydreams and fantasies
After the tone,
He'll get back to you.

Eventually.

The scenic route

Poems don't have to be long.
They can take the bypass
And travel to the heart direct.
But sometimes the scenic route
Is more challenging.
The road through the mind
Can be rough and twisted,
But the view at the end
Makes the journey worthwhile.

Rough night

Tired, sore and out of focus,
My eyes sink back and long for sleep.
Heart and thought locked in competition;
Who can run the fastest pace?
And with thunderous ticking,
A neglected clock welcomes the coming storm.

Suicide

Midday,
But the curtains in her room are drawn.
The door is locked.
The girl sleeps on.
Still, she lies upon her bed,
Rapt in total silence;
Dead.
On the floor an empty bottle,
A few scattered pills.
No note.
No explanation.
Just another suicide,
And only God knows why.

Elaine Fogarty

Into the grey

Choices are the curse of older years
And get worse as time moves on.
Having to choose between this and that,
Think, which one? And either, or.
It's never going to be simple.
There is no black and white.
There is no solid yardstick
On which to measure wrong and right.
There is only more confusion,
And bigger and bigger stakes,
And the feeling you're going to regret it -
Which ever decision you make.
Black and white isn't the answer.
You need to step into the grey;
Hold your breath and quietly listen,
To hear what your heart has to say.

Workday blues

With a ring from my alarm clock,
I rise into the day.
I work; I eat; I sleep.
I let my life waste away.
I travel the same road every morning:
Repetitive and dull.
I wish; I hope; I dream,
For a life that's rich and full.

In too deep

Selfishly clinging
To what is not mine.
Fearfully watching
The passage of time.
Ignoring the consequences,
Of which I'm aware;
I pretend to myself
That I simply don't care.
So much to gain.
Twice as much to lose.
I struggle to justify
The path I choose.

Afterwards

Hospitals and doctors.
Photographs and forms.
All kinds of medication.
Phone calls and reports.
Loneliness and depression.
Guilt mixed with relief.
Anger mixed with sympathy.
A numbness:
Disbelief.
Long waits and long discussions.
Lots of well-meaning advice.
Depression.
Anger.
Worry.
Long days and longer nights.

Embrace

Bless'd, restful sleep.
For these hours of soft embrace,
Weary spirits thank you.

Unclear

Birthdays – days like any other,
Except today I felt so alone.
Neglected, dismissed and forgotten.
Another year gone by;
Not even a card to acknowledge it.
I felt the comfort of others,
But your absence cut deeply.
Lately you've been distant.
Foolishly, today I expected more.
New job? New friends? New needs?
To me your reasons are unclear,
But a friendship of so many years
Should not have died so brutally.

Tradition

Our hero John was a happy lad,
Never known to frown.
That is at least, until the day
He moved to Portadown.
He'd been out with girls from Antrim,
Lisburn and Belfast.
But when he moved to this fair town,
He fell in love at last.
He first saw her at a night club,
"Kings" on a Thursday night.
She was an absolute beauty,
An angel in his sight.
Whilst at the bar he stared at her,
Buying a fortune in beer,
And when she finally spoke to him,
He froze with sudden fear.
There was a little conversation,
And then a dance or two.
They made a date and kept it,
And then another few.
Well, one thing led to another:
Cupid spread his wing,
And before he knew his own mind,
John was buying her a ring.
The poor lad was delighted,
Thinking of the day;
Blissfully ignorant of tradition,
He didn't know our ways.
No one thought to warn him,
No one wanted to.
Why spoil their chance of having fun,
By telling what they'd do.
Three days before the wedding
John arrived at work.
He hoped he'd have a quiet day,
But he was out of luck.
The office was like a ghost town;
No one anywhere,
He walked into the storeroom
And there he got a scare.
With a bang the door slammed behind him;
There was nowhere left to run.
His mates were ready for him.

Ready for their fun.
Cornered at last, he had to give in.
They pulled him to the floor.
Mary and Kathryn held him down,
Others stripped him to the core.
First they took his shirt and tie,
His very socks and shoes.
He did his best to struggle free,
But there was little he could do.
With a little extra manpower,
The trousers came off with ease.
But they decided to leave him something,
Just in case he'd freeze.
All his clothes were bundled up
And thrown into a box,
Then to poor John's horror,
They produced a low cut frock.
They tore the skirt to half its length,
And got rid of both the sleeves,
Then pulled it over john's head
With one almighty heave.
As if that wasn't quite enough,
The girls came to the fore.
They covered his face in make up
And padded the dress he wore.
They stood and looked at John and sighed.
Something wasn't right . . .
They added a bit more padding
And stood back to inspect.
John wished that he could disappear.
He ran towards the door.
But they weren't about to let him go,
For they had more in store.
Everyone helped to carry him,
Out into the yard.
They tied him to a trailer,
And covered him in flour.
They sprayed him with cheap perfume,
And threw and egg or two,
Washed him down with a bucket of water,
And thought what else to do.
It was drawing near to lunchtime,
There were people everywhere.
So they drove the car and trailer out
To let them stand and stare.
The minutes passed like hours,

Then John's heart began to pound.
Someone had suggested
That they drive around the town.
Everyone turned and laughed
As John went slowly by.
He was getting so embarrassed,
He wished that he could die.
All his workmates drove behind him,
Sounding their horns non-stop.
Little kids stood and jeered.
Little old ladies died of shock.
Lunchtime traffic didn't help,
John gave up in despair.
Especially when they reached St. Marks
And he saw the Rector there.
John could have sworn he saw him laugh,
Though he didn't like to say.
But how would he look him in the face,
When they met on Saturday?
Twice round the town then back at last;
John was never so relieved.
Getting married in Portadown he thought,
Wasn't as simple as it seemed.
He went and had a shower,
And thought he'd be all right.
Then he suddenly remembered...
His stag party tomorrow night!
He sat down by the lockers,
Mates all around,
And wondered why he fell in love,
With a girl from Portadown.

Ode to the single

You're gone;
Banished forever from our balcony.
Now there are rows and rows of double seats;
Rows and rows of back row seats.
Double seats for couples, and they're pleased.
They don't miss your tiny awkward curving back.
They don't miss your hard unyielding arm.
Some of them can't even remember you.
But you've lost a lot of friends in leaving;
People who could watch a film alone
And hide, inconspicuous in your care.
Now they sit drowning in huge blue seats;
Seats that remind them of their loneliness,
And display it for the world.

Expectations

Arriving in the season of good intentions,
The new-born year is christened 'Hope'.
A new beginning nurtured in celebration
And showered with gifts of promises.
Very soon he learns the disappointment of reality.
By the age of Summer
He is weary with responsibility.
By the age of Winter
He is content to rest.
By the old, old age of Christmas
He can smile
And know he's done his best.
With the last stroke of midnight he slips away
Into the realm of memory.
Then,
Into a world of expectation,
Is born another to take his place.

Questions

If the road had been wetter, or the cars going faster,
Or the seat belts just not worn?
If the car had been older, or smaller, or lighter,
Or the brakes just not up to form?
So many questions the mind can raise,
And with them such emotions flow.
Sprains and bruises eventually heal.
But will the bad dreams go?

Lottery

Like a child
Forgotten by Santa Claus,
I sit staring at my ticket.
What's wrong with my numbers?
Is that machine deliberately ignoring them?
After a whole year of Christmas
My stocking is still empty,
And I'm still waiting.

To make a circle

New friends,
Faceless friends,
Friends across the sea.
New friends?
Fun friends?
Friends who care about me?
New friends?
Pen friends?
How many will there be?
New friends?
Real friends?
Time can only see.

Because I do

One pencil, three pens,
Red, black and blue,
Always these, only these;
Nothing else will do.
Millimetre square,
Ordered and neat,
Everything in place:
Rituals complete.
Notes – no spaces,
How it should be,
Continuous stream,
No gaps for me.
Rules everywhere,
Correct, tidy, adjust:
I have no choice,
Comply I must.
Checking doors twice,
As I pass through;
Loved ones are safe
Because I do.
Makes little sense
To you, I know,
But this is how
Things have to go.
I do these things,
For safety's sake,
For fear of loss,
Each hour awake.

Secrets

If I told you of secret places,
You'd stop me in my tracks.
If I told you then of secret things,
You'd make me give them back.

Once made they can't be unmade:
My plans now are simple facts.
I think about them often,
No compelling need to act.

Secrets are my safety net,
And so my thoughts attract,
But I may never use them –
At least while hope's intact.

The long night

Here I am again.
On my own.
Night fell hours ago and so did the silence.
Television doesn't make good company,
But it's all I have tonight.
The clock ticks louder and louder,
Counting the minutes 'til daylight.

It's painful being so lonely,
When you have to pretend to be alright.

Reality

Are dreams just an illusion?
Just a stillborn hope of reality?
Sometimes a dream can be so vivid
That it pours over into the morning.
The feelings I'm left with are real.

Are dreams just an illusion?
I'm not so sure.

Workstation

Same screen, same task...
Blurring beyond focus,
Spinning with psychedelic fervour.
My subconscious tramples over it,
Refusing to give it credence.
Half an hour and yet no further.
One hundred disjointed thoughts
Scramble for attention
And time is lost in the confusion.

Three hours

I thought at first to write a poem,
To bemoan the early hour,
To wake so soon after sleep arrived,
Seemed cruel; tasted sour.
My eyes ache still and long for rest.
My mind is wide awake.
A day destined to be difficult,
More challenges still makes.
But rise I will, and thank the hour,
For though an early morning call,
And though I face my mind's assault,
At least I woke at all.

Elaine Fogarty

The switch

Let's be hypothetical
And talk about the switch.
If it were placed before me now,
My outstretched hand would twitch;
My life in balance quickly weighed.
My jumbled thoughts would race,
Then happily I'd leave it be.
My unique path to pace,

Why erase my bipolar life?
It's what has made me 'me'.
It has taken years to realise,
That 'me' is good to be.

Tattoo

Today,
I have this little butterfly.
It rests upon my arm.
It quietly reminds me
To resist self harm.
Tomorrow
Weakness may just kill it,
But today it lives in hope.
My little temporary tattoo,
Simply helps me cope.
Right now,
I don't care if you see it.
I don't care if you ask.
I'm so tired of hiding illness;
So sick of wearing masks.

The night that almost was

The night that could have been,
The night that almost was,
The night that never happened,
Never was, because...
A quiet, gentle whisper
Undermined enticing calls,
Spoke yet again of love and life,
Forced forming plans to stall.
The night that could have been,
The night that almost was,
The night that never happened,
Slips away, as never was.

Blessed

Because I am the way I am,
Because I struggle so,
I've been blessed in helping others:
I understand the lows.
I've been there, bought the T-shirt.
I've courted death and won.
My struggle is so worth it,
If I can help but one.

Belief

As I believe in Heaven,
So must I believe in Hell.
As I believe in Almighty God,
Then Satan must exist as well.
Without evil we can know no good;
Without darkness, know no light.
Without chaos we can know no peace;
Without challenge, climb no heights.
As I believe in the grace of God,
A simple truth must be -
I must believe in Satan,
For He believes in me.

Tickets

I've got my lucky tickets
And I'm waiting now to see
If they'll pick the proper numbers
And give a prize to me.
I'd really love some whiskey,
In fact any alcohol,
But I'd settle for some smellies
Or some vouchers for the mall.
Maybe some yummy chocolates
Or flowers inside a pot.
The table is starting now to bow
Under weight of the whole lot.
Biscuits, bags and boxes.
I hope there's a prize for me.
I'll sit here and guard my tickets
And then later on I'll see.

Connection

Share the darkness,
Share the silence.
That's all I ask today.
Unconditional connection.
No questions.
Not today.

Hedonism and self-loathing.

An intimate and timeless language,
Is heard without a sound:
Whispered promises understood,
When chocolate is around.
The hedonistic smell and taste,
Snuff out all painful thought.
Melting and transforming,
Troubles turning then to nought.
Like some illicit rendezvous,
We meet, and gorge, until,
Primal desire is sated,
And all the world is still.
And rising from this union,
Guilt - palpable and bold,
Merging with self-loathing;
Addiction claims a tighter hold.

Elaine Fogarty

140 or less

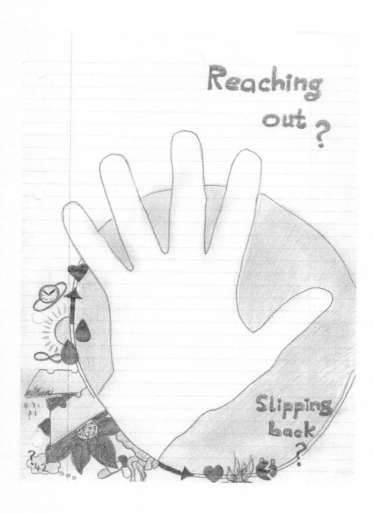

Elaine Fogarty

140-1
The morning skies hang heavy, wrapped in seamless grey. Were they not pregnant with hope and joy, I'd throw this day away.

140-2
The words "I'm fine" are forever tainted, because lies saturate them and fear lurks in their shadow.

140-3
The butterfly is fading, the lines below it too, but cutting works so very well – what else is there to do?

140-4
I only have fine scars; I never cut that deep, but I have dark and detailed plans, and secrets still to keep.

140-5
Should my right hand be timely steeled to do the deed, my weak and conflicted left could scarcely follow through.

140-6
The other day, the thought of suicide crept into my mind... I beat the crap out of it and kicked it back out again. !!!

140-7
Rest now, tear, upon my cheek, and make no rally call. Bring not forth your many friends, but thank them one an' all.

140-8
We all have an inner poet that braves the rapids and guides us to calmer waters.

140-9
Were I a Greek player upon the stage, I could scarcely wait to lower the mask a moment and secretly share truth with the audience.

140-10
Weary eyes so beg to close that sleep could scare refuse. And, so to bed, where mind and soul conspire to paint new truth.

140-11
Into that place between wakeful thought and blessed sleep creeps nightly the image that will not fade: it's part of me now.

140-12
Hidden things and hidden thoughts, wrapt up in secret dreams.
Precious plans hide carefully, and in plain sight, remain unseen.

140-13
Just because they're shallow, doesn't mean there is less pain. Just
because they're hidden, doesn't mean she's safe again.

140-14
The cat lies in her little hammock as midnight creeps close by,
snoring in contentment as I heave a jealous sigh. To bed. To bed.

140-15
I've thought about it many times: the note, and what to say, but
lately thoughts are redirected, as they cry out. 'Not today.'

140-16
I'd settle for a comma, perhaps parentheses, but I'm stuck with a
feckin' period – I so hate days like these!

140-17
Many of us have a plan, once made can't be un-made. The trick is
counting each new day its use can be delayed.

140-18
Smile today at a stranger, what harm could it really do? Your smile
could lift a despairing heart, and lift your spirit too.

140-19
It visits daily – often so fleeting as to melt away again before an
image burns into my mind – the thought, gone before I can even
think.

140-20
The flood gates creak under pressure and I hold my breath in
anticipation of the coming storm.

Meditations

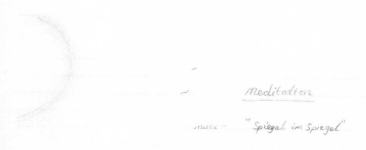

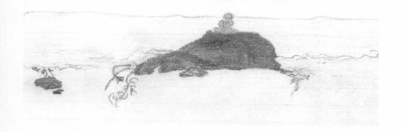

Elaine Fogarty

Communion

Tonight I lie in darkness and gaze into the soft glow of firelight. The initial flurry of yellow soon subsiding, I focus on the soothing drum-like sound. A few resilient sparks linger and cling lightly to the layered soot behind, until finally, even they succumb to the updraft and are gone. Flakes of loose soot still quiver on the edge of the flames – just out of reach – and, like the fire itself, they seem for a moment alive. Ironic, really, that such life, warmth and beauty should be born of the doubly dead tree. Pale yellow gives way to hot blues and soon the emerging white of charcoal scar. There's a beauty there – as if the cracks and lines try to impart their story; for a brief moment I'm lost in their silent tale and witness the seedling's journey. How old were you? Where did you stand? How many birds and animals took shelter in your care? How many lovers rested in your shade or children played among your branches? What did you look like with a blanket of snow or the glow of autumn's glory? How has the world changed around you? What have you seen? What do you know? Even as the flames dance around the log, the driving wind-beat continues, slower yet distinct among the cracks and hisses. Like a slowing pulse it persists – resigned and even content in its tone. A growing amount of smoke rises from the underside and, as it escapes, I fancy it the spirit of the tree and wish it well. Closing my eyes, I drift to sleep with the warmth still brushing my face and its quiet lullaby in my ears. I am no longer alone.

Dusk

Today I stood for over half an hour with my head tilted above the rooftops. I stopped in the street to watch the birds come home to roost. Swarming in bigger and bigger numbers they flew as if following some invisible yet intricate pattern – beautiful. Coming together, staying together, working together – how? Why? More and more of them, and soon I felt like I was up there too, experiencing each swoop and turn for myself. It felt good. When I looked back to the street I realised I'd been the only one watching; the world busied itself around me. Had I imagined its beauty? Had it not been wonderful? Why had no one else noticed? Why did no one else care? They probably had thought me crazy as I stood there, frozen in my private moment of peace. That doesn't trouble me. I see a lot of things others don't seem to see.
These birds were flying like music.

Elaine Fogarty

Walking meditation

"I would scarce have strength to walk this earth, were it not for God's grace pushing gently back with encouragement, every step I take."

I slipped out of the office and down into the warehouse, walking slower and slower as I approached the fire exit door leading to the back loading yard. The warmth of the sun hit my face with intensity as the door swung open and the yard glistened with bejewelled puddles after the recent rain. The birds among the trees and surrounding hedges sang contentedly, and the air tasted so good. It was just a yard like any other, but it was beautiful. With my phone in my jeans pocket and the earphones in, the 'Amazing Grace' album was playing – a whole album featuring one of my all-time favourite hymns in many different arrangements. It played out a gentle rhythm for me as I slowed my pace to match and began to trace the perimeter of the yard, the car park and driveway. Time didn't really much register as I walked, because I became so focused on the music, on my breath and the placement of each individual step. A meditative walk is all about mindfulness. Nothing is without significance. About halfway round I noticed the ground itself pressing back as I pressed down – the hard, hard tarmac gently rebounded and its energy passed to me. There was a definite connection and, given my frame of mind and the music I was listening to, I recognised at once that this was God's way of connecting with me, of helping me. Our walk together in the yard today taught me that God's grace has always been there to support me.

Portstewart

The tip of the pencil taps rhythmically down on the paper; my right hand grasping it lightly and then releasing it repeatedly as I stare vacantly at the computer. My left hand props up my heavy head and, feeling quite ignored, the text on screen begins to soften into abstract patterns and yet I continue to stare. My mind is somewhere else, but even the closing of my eyes fails to summon a clear picture of exactly where: there is a sense of security and comfort as I nestle into the silence and become part of the unnamed emptiness – here, but not here. I can feel the lift and roll of my ribcage as my breath begins to deepen and slow and then, from the heavy mists of nothingness, comes the elusive image. I'm in Portstewart, on a day like any other, save the briskness of the sea winds and the crashing of the sea against ragged rocks in front of me. The sound is hypnotic and the dancing foam is truly beautiful to watch. The seagulls' call adds melody to the music of the sea. Hubby and I have always loved this spot; the bench below us so well used it has almost begun to mould itself into the shape of our two bodies, Hubby sitting upright in the corner and me snuggling in like a child listening to a bed time story. Right now, now is all there is. We have nowhere to be, nothing to do, no responsibilities to tend... we can sit here for hours... in fact, we often have. The scent of sea air is momentarily overpowered by the smell of freshly cooked chips; we enjoy a bag full each and they seem better than any ever eaten before. Indulgently heavy on salt and dripping in vinegar, the chips are cooked to perfection and we tuck in straight away, glad of the heat offered up by the little paper bag of yumminess. A few sea gulls patrol the pathway and wall around us, willing us to drop a chip so they can also feast, but we selfishly deny them their prize. The cold evening air rolls in as we eat, but we are in no rush to move on; conversation gives way to comfortable silence and we look out to sea together, united in our appreciation of its beauty and lost in our own daydreams. And so begins the daydream within a daydream and I am doubly lost.

Meditation on a tree

I am so very old and stand contentedly by a riverbank, bathed in autumn glory and nurtured by the running waters. I am at once all things – I am the tree, the water, the air, the songbirds in the leaves, everything, the entire world; all at once and yet in a place beyond space and time. Calmness washes over me as water washes over the exposed roots. I am at home. I am at rest. My breath disappears into the rhythm of the universe itself and I am lost. All that matters is here. There is timelessness, balance and, above all, peace. I am the tree, and sepulchred lie the seeds of spring itself. Autumn will pass. Winter will pass. Spring and summer will erupt into joyous abundance whether their effort is noticed or not. I stand witness to it all – to all change – all seasons – all time – all life.

{The sketch shows the aged tree standing right on the riverbank itself with its autumn leaves almost all shed. Its twisted roots protrude from the clay. Vibrant leaves lie scattered on the grass or floating in the river – one is caught mid air.}

Elaine Fogarty

Spiegel im Spiegel

It was my first night on the ward and I suddenly craved fresh air. I needed to feel it, to taste it, to let it wash away all my uncertainties. Having come to rely on it, panic rose quickly when it was denied me. All I needed was five minutes outside. I needed to escape the lifeless air; the stale air that locked doors and sealed windows had created. I hadn't realised how much I relied on our time together until I could no longer claim it. My protestations having gone unheard, I made my way back to my bed, drew the curtain partially round and, with that beautiful piece of music playing softly in my earphones, I began to mediate – an old skill resurrected. I emerged from that seashore almost half an hour later; there were a few tears, but they were not sad ones. I felt calm and refreshed, and the ward around me didn't look quite so scary. (The moon seemed bigger as it cast its rays across the velvety sea. The waves, in deference to my needs, crept ashore in time with my own breath. Fresh, cool, salty sea air filled my lungs, and there on that rock I drank in the sensation of freedom and peace. I felt the air brush my skin like a lover's caress and my hair swept gently back as if to follow and capture it. A few moments later I walked along the shoreline; night surf tickled my toes as I walked. My footprints pressed into the damp sand and it pressed back as if to encourage my journey.)

{Half the page is the beach scene from the mediation. In the centre a silhouette of me sitting cross-legged on a large rock and the calm sea stretches out to infinity. The moon is large and to the left of the sky. The eye is drawn to two birds in flight.}

Rain – a meditation

The rain clings like transparent Matrix code, broken lines running down my bedroom window. Behind it the warm, orange glow of a nearby streetlight captures my attention for what seems like an eternity, and as I stare at it the sound of the rain intensifies. It's heavy rain, the type that saturates the small grass lawns and spills out onto the driveways, runs down the roads without taking time. The wind tries to make itself heard periodically, but I barely hear it above the hypnotic sound of large raindrops hitting the roof just above my head. The bedside clock that would normally scream to draw attention to itself still ticks but, oh, so quiet in my perception. All I hear is rain – and it speaks to me. I wish I could be out there with my old friend. I've shared more raw emotion with the rain over

72

the years than with anyone I've ever met. Hugs are magical and healing, but a walk in the rain is a communion of spirit – a walk in the rain is a deeply powerful thing to those open to its influence. I love the rain. My window is open and spots of rain begin to creep inside, calling me. Oh, how little it would take for me to accept that invitation, but the hour grows late and I must content myself with its music as I wait for restful sleep. I close my eyes and imagine myself walking the street, allowing the rain to wrap itself around me, and smile as minutes slow like deep time and I feel understood – I feel at peace.

Elaine Fogarty

Journal entries

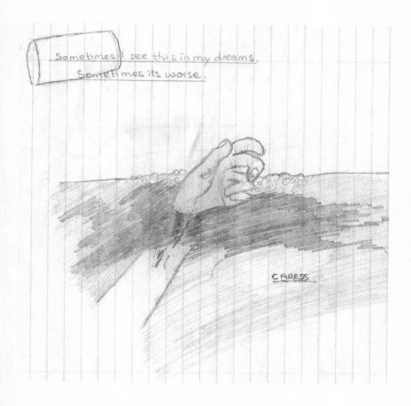

Elaine Fogarty

These surviving journal entries span almost 30 years. Most were originally loose and crumpled pages, scribbled in pencil and interlaced with sketches. I've presented the transcripts as close to the original content as possible. They are laid out non-sequentially and have not been unnecessarily edited. Where sketches, charts etc were present, there is a notation below the main body of text.

A quivering quark

"This evening I am strangely calm, yet a wake of uneasiness follows me wherever I go. This calm belies the seriousness of my true state – I am just a quivering quark away from totally breaking down. I am scared. I don't want to ruin next week's holiday for everyone but I can't see how to keep it together long enough to carry the holiday through to an uneventful end. My stronger self reminds me that my ability to recognise what's going on is itself a good thing, my calmness in the face of ill-timed problems to be applauded. I can't see it... it's unnatural to be this calm... something is seriously wrong... pressure is quietly building... with explosive force, something may soon give and my depression will ride the pressure wave until it forces shutdown: there may be no stopping it."

Hols tomorrow

"Tomorrow morning I am heading away on a family holiday. I spent the better part of this evening gathering stuff and packing bags. Not that fond of the job, but it usually falls to me when we travel. Fair enough I suppose because Hubby does all the driving – can't complain. As my depression has been eating at me for a while now, it will be nice to get away somewhere quiet and slow-paced. We have a little cottage booked so we can really do as little or as much as we like – when we like. Perfect. It should do me the world of good they say – I hope they are right.

In the back of my mind though, my best mate's wedding – tomorrow – while we are on holiday. How much does that suck??? Totally gutted that I am going to miss it but when we were told the date it was already too late to cancel the trip. Hoping that some kind person will message me a couple of photos at least. I'll be thinking of them all day and sending every good wish it is in me to send."

Note

"I'm sorry to have left you like this. I love you but I can't stay, I ca"

{Neatly written on a lined A5 page but never finished. The page crumpled and intended for the bin}

Tired

"I'm so tired, but I just can't sleep. My mind just won't shut up! There's a voice in my head telling me that tomorrow is a waste of time and that I'm a waste of space. She says there's no point in trying any more – I'll never fit in. She says it would just be better, easier, if I didn't wake up. She's right. She's making sense – of course she would, because she's me. I'm the voice inside my own head, talking to myself, trying to convince myself that life isn't going to get any better – it's like me talking to me – how f**ked up is that?"

{Scribbled diagonally across a file block page, filling it. Almost unreadable}

Whisper

"There is a constant stinging sensation coming from my arm. There is no pain, just this whisper reminding me of recent cuts. I won't go into detail because it would be unfair to risk triggering someone else, but it is what it is ... I cut ... and somehow it made everything seem a little better, as it always does. I'm going into work soon and I've chosen to wear a long sleeved top – it gives me options – three inch square white dressings are not easy to conceal but then they know about my 'issues' in work which means I shouldn't have to worry about covering up on such a warm and clammy day. I guess I'll play it by ear when I get in. It's going to be a very long day in work today because I am genuinely in no state to get anything done – my mind will not be on the job at hand, that's for sure... But in I go because I'm thinking it's better than sitting the eight hours alone with my thoughts"

Deceitful and dangerous

"This morning I contacted my CPN and asked to move our appointment forward, because I had something important to discuss. My logic told me this was the right thing to do, but if it's so right why am I sitting here this evening without the first clue on what

I'm going to say? Why do I feel a little anxious? As I sat in the car that evening, I knew I was getting worse, I knew I was in crisis. I knew it was real. I knew they were deceitful and dangerous but I was finding it harder and harder to push away the dark thoughts. A growing part of me believed there was nothing left worth living for and was reviewing plans. My instinct told me that if I rang the CMHT I'd find myself back on the ward, because of this I could recognise what a bad place I was in. I suppose going back on the ward would have been no bad thing, and to my credit, I remained aware enough to still be comparing options; my little CBT voice was still chipping away. In the end I went back to the source and made contact with Hubby; he of course got me home and helped me feel safe and loved again. The desperate suicidal thinking is gone now as quickly as it appeared, supplanted by a vague uneasiness. I think I made the right choice, I still need to talk about it though – can't ignore it out of existence – after all, Saturday was the first 'suicidal crisis' in about six years. I'm somewhat nervous of the speed and intensity with which it manifested but it IS gone. I was a little unsettled for a while afterwards but I'm ok. I need to let her know what happened though. But I still don't have a clue what to say. How do I talk about how embarrassed I feel now, or how stupid, how weak? What are the words to describe the lingering fear of what might have been?"

Distinctly anxiety free

"Today, not a lot happened. It has been an entirely unremarkable day in every way but one – today I had my first 'normal' work day in ages. The work came in. The work got done. I stayed calm and prioritised and found lunch time and home time both rolled round without extensive clock-watching and paper shuffling. I'm as chuffed as a little steam train climbing a mountain. I've pretty much re-established my routine and just playing a little catch-up to get things as they should be. I am so impressed with my concentration today as well – even managed to investigate and solve some irritating queries. If work is getting easier that means I'll soon be on the mend again – my mood may be beginning to settle again. Yes – I am tired. Still, what a difference I've seen ... what a difference I've felt. Sometimes the absence of an emotion is as notable as its presence and today was distinctly anxiety free. Most importantly, I didn't once today feel the urge to self harm (well unless you count the deliciously fun task of peeling off scabs – that's normal right? Other people do that too right?)"

Caress

"One second, less than one second... That's all it took. It jumped into my mind and for a split second I smiled. I can still feel the warm water and the tiny bubbles breaking against my skin. But all I remember about the blood is how it made me smile. It was back. The image popped into my mind uninvited and was gone as quick – at the time I smiled. It was familiar – comforting – but now when I think about it, I'm noticing how uncomfortable it makes me feel – That couldn't be me? I mean... It couldn't... could it? Oh God, it felt so real... But when I pictured it this morning and thought to draw it, what the hell prompted me to label it 'caress'? Is this really me? Sometimes I see this in my dreams as well. Sometimes it's worse."

{The sketch is better than my usual ability, very detailed. From elbow to fingers, the arm lies limply at the surface of water. A three inch deep cut runs vertically along the vein and lots of blood flows from it creating a floating surface pool. This is the sketch I showed my GP when trying to explain the stuff I was living with}

Pens are too slow

"Someone asked me today how come I could write when I was feeling so rotten. The simple answer is that it is a coping mechanism that acts a bit like a release valve. I sit down with my family, my CPN or my psychiatrist and I often have difficulty articulating my thoughts, but when I write it all somehow flows – it's the same with poetry – you know it's working when it sort of starts to write itself and takes you in a direction you didn't think you wanted to go. If I write on paper I have to use pencil because pens are too slow and sometimes even a nicely rounded pencil tip can't move as fast as the jumbled outpouring of thoughts. I'm by no means a perfect touch typist but I have enough speed to make my laptop a perfect tool. Finally a journal that is actually legible."

Me vs Me

"It's after one – Part of me desperately wants to sleep but part of me wants to write the jumbled thoughts down so they will go away. I'm conflicted, but that's nothing new; these guys have been arguing for days now. Friday I was low and unsettled – part of me was calm and stoical, part of me was concerned. Saturday the bottom fell out of my world – part of me saw nothing worth living for, part of me saw the whole world. Sunday I looked for a way to come to terms with what had happened – part of me wanted to ring in a couple of sick days, part of me saw no need. And so it went on, particularly with phone calls, phone calls to ask for help. Saturday, and every day since, I lifted the phone to call my Community mental health team; part of me needed to talk, part of me didn't know what to say. I'd lift the phone then set it down I'd start to ring but then hang up. I'd get through but decide not to say anything, not to leave a message. Part of me was confident it was all over and done with, that there was no harm in talking, part of me was afraid it would see me back on the ward. I don't want that. I rang again today. I did not leave a message. I feel remarkably settled today. I'm not even feeling negative. Bizarre as it sounds, I sense the episode of depression has now passed. What happened was an isolated response to an isolated and quite spontaneous event. It has passed too. Part of me wants to move on now, part of me is scared I won't be able to until I talk to my CPN about it all. Perhaps I should have left a message? Perhaps I will."

Surrender to the rain

"I made it into work today after much inner debate – considering the merits of social interaction and distraction over silence and isolation. Distraction won and only half an hour past my start time, I walked sleepily through the office door. Still not totally convinced, I lingered over a coffee then buried myself in repetitive data entry. Anything requiring complex thought was left in the tray, but it was still quite a productive day I think. Things are difficult right now and there seems to be a constant stream of problems, issues and irritations to ensure I don't find a fast route out of this current depression. I can barely think straight and everything around me seems to be going wrong – not wrong in a negative perception kind of way but the kind of wrong that would challenge any regular Joe. On the way home from work the car exhaust decided to detach its rear box and the sound of its banging would perhaps during other episodes, have pushed me over the edge – the words camel straw and back come to mind. Something weird happened though. I went all calm instead. How can I explain it? Ever been caught in sudden heavy rain whilst out walking? With no shelter in sight there very soon comes a point where you surrender to the rain – you are so wet you just can't get any wetter – so why fight it? It was a bit like that. I've bottomed out now. My mood hasn't changed. There has been no sudden shift of polarisation. I have just realised that it's not going to get any worse. That's something at least."

The dream

"From the corner of my garden, in the corner of my mind came the haunting and incessant sound of a cat meowing – not just any cat, but my dearest Krissy. With me for over twelve years and then cruelly lost – my dreamy instinct knew that it is somehow her. She could always sense when I felt low and would come to me, softly purring and gently kneading with her paws as she pressed in close and reminded me that I didn't have to face it alone. Before anyone else, she was always there; she just knew. The sound draws me close and the dream makes perfect sense of what I find as I tip open the loose lid of a blue spotted cool bag – three tiny overly fluffy jet black little kittens with large endearing eyes – three Krissy kittens – all at once the same cat I had virtually hand reared – all her. Three darling Krissys all looking up at me in recognition and asking to be lifted. I gathered them into my arms and carried them inside. My dream swept us in an instant to my favourite chair and once again I felt the healing purr reverberate around me, through me – my world closed in and denied the pain access – I felt a peace I hadn't felt in months. Two lay curled in my lap and one climbed up to my shoulder and nestled into my neck. All was lost to the mists of the dream but my own soft smile and that familiar sound. In a dream within a dream I drifted off, content and unafraid. I awoke into the real world what seemed only seconds later. I was dazed and confused. As my eyes adjusted to the 3am glow of street lights outside, I began to recall flashes, disjointed images and rushes of emotion as I slowly untangled the dream from reality. They were gone. She was gone. I cuddled into the quilt and noted a tear hanging tentatively on the corner of my eye. As this single tear rolled down on to my cheek I realised that I was smiling and I silently thanked her for finding a way back to me when I needed her. Who's to say that dreams aren't real? Such distinctions are beyond our understanding."

Alone again

"In less than half an hour Hubby is going out. This is a pre-existing thing, he told me about it last week, I knew about it. Thing is, when he mentioned it again an hour or so ago, a wave of panic rushed through me. He was going out and I'd be alone in the house. I don't want to be alone tonight, not even for a couple of hours, because I really can't trust myself just yet. I know that but I don't want to admit it. It's so hard to shake all that stuff that filled my Saturday. I don't want to be alone tonight because I'm distracted when around other people, doing stuff together, going places together – those unwelcome thoughts can't find their way in. I don't want to be alone tonight because I'm anxious and scared. Ridiculous, I'm 45 and scared of sitting alone in my own house for 2/3 hours – it makes me feel stupid. I've set myself a goal of getting back to work Wednesday so I suppose I need to step outside my comfort zone tonight if I stand any chance of being at my desk midweek."

Damn radio

"I picked a really bad day to come back to work....
Turns out its 'World mental health day.'
The radio has done little but talk at length about suicide and depression.
Damn radio!!"

The worst mistake I've made all year

"So, I was thinking about how I wanted to talk to my psychiatrist about OCD – and more specifically, whether or not my slightly unusual 'habits' are indeed a presentation of just that. My next review appointment is due before Christmas which is ideal but the more I thought about it, the more I realised – after 6 years' working with him without mentioning this, I was going to need significantly more than a standard 20 mins consultation to suddenly reveal my little secret. The better part of this morning was spent composing a letter to introduce the idea and accompany printed copies of all those notes I had prepared to try and fully explain it all. It's an unconventional approach, certainly proactive, but it serves both of us well by giving him time to review the information and decide how best to proceed when we do meet face to face. At least, that's what I'm telling myself; it may turn out to be the worst mistake I've made all year! The envelope is going in the post tomorrow morning and, good idea or bad, it will be too late. I've kept this to myself for a long time and I'm feeling a little exposed now that it's going out in the open. I need to talk to him about this but when the letter arrives naming the date, I'm going to be more nervous than I was during the wait for O- and A-level results all those years ago."

Custard creams and denial

"Last night was one of those – one of those nights that we never talk about. This morning it's coffee, TV and conversation about what's for lunch – neither of us want to talk about what could have happened last night – what really came so close to happening. It's custard creams, coffee and denial. It should be talked about but it won't be. Fair enough, you think, maybe next time – but what if next time there is no morning, no coffee and biscuits? What if next time the house is shrouded in silence and it's too late for conversation? The 'what-ifs' dance around my mind like playful faeries but I can't indulge them; it's too dangerous."

Not keeping score... but

"I've just come home from an evening wedding party and these sorts of functions do not normally mix well with my social anxiety. I never know until I walk into the main room how it's going to go – tonight's scores went a bit like this....
Entering, I was able to swallow down the creeping anxiety. Score 1 Elaine. I even smiled and laughed as I hugged the beautiful bride. Score 1 Elaine. I sat in a group near the bar rather than back to the wall in a corner. Score 1 Elaine. I talked away most of the evening. Score 2 Elaine. I got very anxious picking my way through the crowds on the way to the toilets alone. Score 1 Social anxiety. I had a private moment of panic when I got lost in the maze of busy corridors and rooms. Score 2 Social anxiety. I made it on my own to the toilets and back again later in the evening. Score 3 Elaine. I mingled. Score 2 Elaine. And the final scores... Social anxiety 3 Elaine 10. It's so good to come out on top for once – Yay – feeling just a little smug."

Can they see?

"Sometimes I wonder about it...I mean...is it that they don't see or they don't care? Sometimes I wonder if anyone will notice if I wear the same clothes for 3 even 4 days...Do they see the unwashed hair and the really bad skin? Bruises cuts and clumsiness? Do they see the sunglasses indoors? Do they understand me when I rattle on? Do they understand me when say nothing? Do they see me sway, scratch, tap, bite at my nails? Do they think it odd that I'm wide awake at 4am? Do they see me panic in crowds or cringe at loud noises? Notice I barely wash? Can they see the swollen red eyes and the lingering tears? Can they hear the deafening silence? Do they see it and yet ignore it – or do they see it and look through it to check I'm still inside at all? I know a lot of this is me...but it's not all I am. My priorities have just shifted that's all...I've more difficult issues to deal with. There's more going on than people see."

Picture this

"Picture this – I'm in a car accident. I've made it out alive but have serious injuries – any one of which could still kill me. I'm in intensive care. I've got the best treatment, my doctor can see the extent of my injuries, and so can everyone else. They're obviously real. They're worried. They wonder what they can do to help. Friends and relatives rally to the bedside with smiles and hugs and all the support needed. Everyone at work sends best wishes, a card and flowers. 'Take all the time you need,' I'm told. 'Just get well. Concentrate on healing. We'll look after everything else.' I may or may not die – but the odds are definitely in my favour. Now picture this – Depression – Oh how I sometimes wish it had been the other way round...
Odds don't feel so good @ my end."

Megaphone

"Why does no one hear what I'm actually trying to say? I feel like I'm shouting at the top of my lungs and I'm ignored, dismissed or treated like a pain in the ass. Someday I'll tire of shouting for help and they'll all stand around discussing how they didn't see it coming and if only they'd known. Not to mention the 'How could she have been so selfish?' No wonder so many people kill themselves. Even when you ask for help, no one hears you. I bet loads of people die thinking 'well you b*st*rds...at least now you know I was telling the truth!' Me – 'I can't take this anymore. I'm so very tired of it all. I've had enough. Live isn't worth living anymore. I wish I'd never been born.' Them – 'She's great. She seems tired. She's over-reacting. She's so moody. Oh for God's sake cheer up. I'm here if you ever need me – just ring. Pull yourself together. You're just chasing attention. She'll be fine. Grow up. You're no fun anymore. She's a bit down. You need to snap out of it. You think you've got problems. No point in asking anymore... she never comes out. Life is tough... get used to it. She's so lazy. Snap out of it. Stop moaning. She's more trouble than she's worth. She hasn't said anything much in a few days...
She must be fine.' ...The ignorance is palpable."

{A4 lined page. Below main text there is a sketch of a tiny stick figure standing on top of a high and precarious pile of blocks, shouting through a megaphone. Speech bubbles come from here and from the crowds of stick figures down at ground level}

Hello

"Wide awake and busy at after 3am these past four nights – well, hello hypomania, haven't seen you in a while!"

Magnifying glass

"So, my CPN says she isn't dismissing the intensity of what happened, but that I need to stop looking at it with my imaginary magnifying glass, trying to understand it, and what it means for my future. She says I have no need to be afraid of it, of myself. She says it was real, yes. It was dangerous, yes. BUT – what I should be focussing on is the way I was able to 'talk myself down'. The ability to consider other options is something I definitely would not have been capable of 6 years ago, maybe even 6 months ago. She says the circumstances and emotions that led to my sudden onset suicidal state were in fact risk factors for anyone – absolutely anyone. I needed to recognise normalcy in my life as my familiar extremes begin to settle. I had nothing to be ashamed of. She told me to take a step back and look at the positives – My reaction to run was actually a normal response, I just took it to an extreme. My 'CBT voice' was saying all the right things and I was able to make good choices. Before making a call for help, I had already looked suicide in the eye and told her I had other arms to embrace me, that she could not have me. I did all that.
I did all that ALONE. She reminded me that I was stronger than I thought and because I had done it once, I could do it again; I had no reason live with the fear of what could have been."

30 years

"As I lie here in bed and let the thoughts think themselves out, a familiar question revisits. 'How the hell did I manage to survive this long?' I've spent almost my entire life hiding stuff and telling lies – no one knew. Why would they? All those times when I was feeling suicidal – no one knew. All those times I was virtually paralysed by anxiety – no one knew. All those times I hid evidence of self harm – no one knew. I was alone in a crowded life and I didn't understand what was happening. I was afraid so I kept my secret. I was scared but I kept fighting. I don't know where I found that strength; I can't believe I'm still here 30 years on!!"

Appointment anxiety

"Thinking about my next appointment. My review appointments at the hospital always fall on a Thursday or a Tuesday – Tuesday, I almost always see my consultant and Thursdays, it's almost always one of his team. I've got used to seeing lots of different faces and I can't say it bothers me, but each has their own style. My consultant is a lovely man and I have total confidence in him; his style is very much 'discuss' rather than 'chat.' I requested that I meet with Dr. M himself this time because that's what I need. I need to discuss what I believe are OCD symptoms; I am hoping to get a dx to explain all the weirdness. He won't mess about – he will tell me straight and then I will know once and for all. The anticipation of this conversation is what makes me keen to attend on Tuesday of next week. The knowledge that I will also have to discuss my recent suicidal state fills me with dread however. I'm conflicted. I tried talking about it. Only a couple believed me. The rest played my experience down and tried to tell me it wasn't really what I thought it was. Realising that talking was a waste of time, I have of late returned to the 'bottle up, smile and avoid' tactic – I can't invest in real conversation with people who won't believe what I tell them. Come Tuesday, I should discuss what happened but I'm scared he will dismiss me as well. No reason to believe that he would, it's just others have let me down. The closer I get to the appointment date, the more anxious I become."

Bubbles and pins

"Apparently bipolar depression isn't a real illness. The conversation started badly and just kept getting worse – I know I said I was ill with depression, but I'm convinced he heard something completely different. Dismissal stung and the inference that I had just been making weak excuses was insulting – I found it hard not to be angry. Things should have been different. Thing is – I feel cheated because I SO want to rant and rave and get all annoyed and sarcastic, truthfully I'd love to, but I can't. I can't because deep down I know he meant no harm – he simply didn't understand. It wasn't his fault. I could have explained it better. I had mentioned my depression before but most people don't understand what that means; 'depression' is a word so tainted by being loosely thrown around that it does little to sum up the cocktail of despair, apathy, confusion and anxiety I'm living with right now. When you feel as delicate as a floating bubble, everything and everyone around you starts to look an awful lot like a pin. I'm oversensitive – I can't expect everyone to understand what bipolar disorder is – what depression is. I shouldn't be so hyper-sensitive. What was I thinking?"

The dam broke

"Colin arrived and I started to tell him about my day and how I was feeling – it all just sorta came out – the silly trivial things as well as the important. I had been anxious before he arrived, but I began to get worse. I got so worked up that I frightened Colin and he fetched a nurse. She came and calmly asked me about it all – the dam broke + it all flooded out – everything – all the stuff I'd needed to say since I'd arrived. I felt better for it and she arranged some changes in my meds to try and help. She listened – the real kind of listened – like we were the only two people there, and she calmly answered all the questions one by one. That was such a help. I felt a stone lighter. This is the kind of support I had been craving. My state has been so unpredictable and coming on to the ward had ramped up the anxiety, but now I felt much calmer. I wish I could remember her name – it annoys me that I can't."

Long distance to travel

"I'm not currently feeling suicidal but I do still think about it from time to time – quite a lot lately in fact, due to recent events. Last night I didn't sleep so well – my mind insistently drew me back to plans made long ago, plans that still stand ready should I ever need them. Little changes and improvements slot into details long decided, and mentally I check off all the seemingly insignificant things that I keep about me until one day they're needed. In a strange way, my secrets, my plans, are comforting and knowing I always have those options available to me gives me the freedom to keep exploring other paths. If all else fails, I know they will be there for me – I don't find this frightening. It shouldn't frighten others. My plans will most likely never be called to action but I will defend them with everything I have because I need them so desperately. There have been times when those carefully laid plans came within minutes of fruition – it was real – they were as real as they could ever be – but it was not their time. Some day their time may yet come, some day they may prove to be all I have left. They are a part of me now. I can't change that. I can't dwell on that. No matter how 'stable' I seem to be or how well I feel, I will never tell anyone my plans. If I do, it will mean they become instantly unuseable – why would I do that to myself after years of developing them? My admission that I have such plans shouldn't scare people: it doesn't mean I'm definitely going to use them. I don't even know that myself. No one knows the future. We walk past fire extinguishers all the time but it doesn't mean we live in constant paralysing fear of raging fire. It might happen – it probably won't. It's hard to explain, but there is a long distance to travel on the journey from thinking about suicide to being resolutely and imminently suicidal."

7.30pm

"7.30 in the evening and I haven't really got out of bed. Fed the cat, went to the toilet and made a sandwich – that's it. Don't think I'd have even made that banana sandwich if my tummy hadn't been rumbling so very loud. I've listened to Classic FM while I lay here and thought + dozed etc. Oh, and I spent about 1½ hours browsing the internet reading random stuff about depression and suicide.

Mum rang to check I was ok – she's the only one who has contacted me. I feel like crap and can't even concentrate to watch TV. Feel very alone. Nothing says go away like curtains drawn and lights out. But yet I'd like some company – someone to share the darkness. No one seems to want to do that – they want to pull me into their world but I'm not ready yet – not today. Help only exists on their terms I guess. No one will risk getting too close, too involved. They can't deal when I'm unwell. Why must I always be expected to climb up the pit wall? Why can't someone just once climb down and sit a while? Headache now from all this writing but at least the pain kills the chatter."

{The sketch takes up a quarter of the A4 page. Concentric circles with various shading to represent a deep and dark pit. Head and arms of a tiny stick figure are just visible at the bottom of the pit.}

A-Z

"Some things go unheard. Sometimes it doesn't matter. And then, sometimes...

"All I want to do is die"
"It would be better for everyone if I wasn't here"
"I can't take this anymore"
"I Dream about death all the time"
"Everyone would be better off without me"

"I've it all figured out"
"God will understand"
"Everyone hates me"
"It's too late now"
"Just leave me alone"
"Maybe I should just kill myself"
"I have nothing to live for"
"My life is a living hell"
"Nobody cares about me"
"I wish it was all over"
"People are so very cruel"
"It's easier to just quit"
"I'd rather die"
"They'll be sorry"
"I've no tears left"
"I am totally unlovable"
"I am so very tired"
"I wish I was dead"
"I shouldn't exist"
"You just don't understand"
ZZzzzz "I wish I could just fall asleep and never wake up""

If they ask...

"My arm has 'marks' on it at the moment – some permanent scars and some healing areas where the skin had been scratched raw; I don't think it looks that bad, it's been a lot worse. I very rarely hide my arms away any more because I'm no longer ashamed of them. I don't wear my 'marks' as a badge of honour announcing allegiance to some misunderstood sub-culture, but I simply allow them to exist. If people see them they see them. If people ask I answer. It is what it is. My self harm is mild on a comparative scale, but still difficult to explain sometimes: today I had to find a succinct way to do it for someone close who was totally unaware of my mental illness and who was using English as her second language. A challenge. It was a few hours ago but if I recall correctly I simply responded to her pointing finger and puzzled query with this... "Oh, no ... it's not that ... I did it myself ... How can I explain? ... Did he tell you about my illness, my mental illness? Well sometimes people who are sick like that, they do this...they self harm... I did this... I self harm too." I needn't have worried – her hug told me she understood."

Empty bottle

"Almost every day it flashes briefly into my mind in some guise or another, but when I cycle into depression it finds purchase in my troubled mind; the word, the image, the plan. Suicide. At times like this it taunts me, confuses me, and erodes my self esteem to the point I can't even trust my own mind. Its menacing presence has shadowed me since my early teens and the first real poem I ever wrote carried its name. I am 41 years old now but that first poem has been engrained in my memory ever since the night it was first scribbled down."

Yoghurt pots

"Promises are like yoghurt pots ... they come with expiration dates. Someone keeps stocking the shelves with different enticing flavours but at the end of the day, they're all just yoghurt and they're all going to end up in the bin because of short shelf life. Splat! Another one splits open and splashes as it hits the bottom of the bin. Another one out of date, another promise gone. I was stupid to think this one was any different to last week's purchases, or the week before. Last week I said I'd had enough; I was done checking the fridge – I mean really, who was I kidding? Fridges don't make things last forever. Nothing lasts forever. I was a fool to believe the advertising. I won't make that mistake again. Even if a steak and pepper sauce flavour yogurt appears in there tomorrow, I'm still not biting, there's just nothing in there for me anymore."

Abruptly ripped

"Today I was full of the joys... up early, full shower and out for a walk. A short time later though, I started to get really jittery for no apparent reason. I decided to meditate. I sat on my bed as it is the place I feel most comfortable in the absence of my own mat in my own house. I left the music playing on low speaker, did some stretches + breathing exercises and then into a REALLY deep meditation – I assumed I'd be left alone. I assumed wrong. A well-meaning hand tapped me on my leg and ripped me abruptly from my meditation. That's bad, even dangerous anyhow, but when I opened my eyes and saw a strange face in what for a moment was a strange place, I freaked. The combination of a broken meditation and the fright knocked me into a real state. I got angry. I shouldn't have for it wasn't his fault – he had only wanted to offer a cup of tea; he had no idea what he had done. A half hour's deep meditation down the drain – I felt worse than when I had started."

Anger masks the pain

"I'm insanely jealous of all those people my Hubby spends time with – his brother, his motorbike pals, all the guys in all those clubs and associations he is involved with. I'm jealous and upset because they take him away from me and I'm a little angry because he can have a social life and I can't. Because I feel so isolated and lonely and feel a sense of entitlement as I watch others enjoy their social lives, I start to get angry at the world, angry at Hubby. That's not right. That's not fair. It's not Hubby's fault that I have social anxiety or that my bipolar illness in one way or another drove people away over the years. It's not his fault that I cling so desperately to our weekends together, that they sometimes feel like my only chance to do nice things, go to nice places; since most of the time it feels like Hubby is all I have, I impose expectations on our weekend time together that are totally unrealistic. I expect it to be perfect and it never is. In one breath I'll say, "Sure, I'll be fine ... go out for a bike run" and then later when I'm alone I start to feel jealous, upset, and angry. I know I shouldn't do it but it just sort of happens. I've made repeated attempts to become more active socially but for the most part they have imploded, each time I withdraw a little more and feel a little more useless and hopeless. I'm not angry at Hubby for getting out there and having a life – I guess I'm really just angry that I can't, I'm angry at myself, at the world. The anger masks the pain."

Climbing a cliff with fingernails

"It's almost lunch time and what I've achieved so far today is to dress and make it to the couch, to check email, Twitter and blog – oh, and accept a parcel from the persistent postman who saw the car parked outside and assumed repeated knocking and ringing would drag me from my bed. As it turns out he was right, but being up isn't all it's cracked up to be. I wasn't sleeping all that time – since I called in to excuse myself from work early in the morning I lay awake just trying to make sense of how I was feeling. There is heaviness about me, slowness, dullness and the dark thoughts are beginning to linger longer when they visit. I've been here many times before yet each time I indulge the same self pity and begin to shut myself off. I'm getting a little better at spotting it and I like to believe I'm getting a little better at coping with it – it is really important that I don't continue what I started this morning – I can't allow myself to shut off completely and withdraw further. My brother in law and his wife are moving house today. My Hubby took the day off to help them. Maybe I should go round, get out, get some air, and be around people even though the thought of it scares me a little? I'm expected to meet with them this evening anyway for a planned celebration – (R) finally finished her course and handed in that dissertation that kept her up to the small hours each night. It's important that I be part of that – it's going to take a massive effort to get out and actually DO something today but I know I have to. I just can't think straight. I feel like crap. GP appointment at 5pm – I didn't request it, he called me in, so I can't bunk off that either as it might be really important. I feel like crawling into bed again and wishing the world away. I feel like self harming to make it all go away but I will get out there and try to be 'as normal as possible' for a couple of hours at least. If you have suffered depression you know what a mammoth task I set myself and how exhausting it will be. If you are lucky enough to read this having never experienced depression, then please try to understand that it's like climbing a cliff with your fingertips whilst all the while tempted to just let go and be done. This is of course made worse when you encounter people who only see a moody pain in the ass who is just attention-seeking and needs to get over herself already. As I said, I have been here before. I have got through it before. I will again. So even though I look a mess and my hair needs washed and my skin is in terrible condition and my eyes are red and puffy and my arm is a mess with 'marks' and I can't think straight and I'm feeling so totally miserable... I can maybe paint on a smile, muster some conversation and pretend for a while that I'm OK – hell – maybe I'll even convince myself."

The mouth's sense of humour

"Sometimes 'dry mouth' isn't actually that dry; sometimes the slightly swollen tongue is caught between the back teeth and the bite triggers a rush of previously elusive saliva. The area is suddenly awash with well-intended moisture, but it is too late – the damage is done – the swollen tongue now boasts a little bite-sized swelling of its own. It will catch easily and irritate with every meal, every conversation, and as the cursing of it still hangs in the air, the saliva once again makes a hasty retreat and gloats as it hides with impunity. It will return only when it loses interest in the game and there is no more fun to be had laughing at the inadequacies of 'saliva replacements' and pastilles that seek to tempt it out of seclusion. The mouth's sense of humour, like itself – seems quite dry."

Is the door sticking?

""Is the door sticking" she said, as I came back into the office. Right there I knew it had finally become too obvious and people were noting the 'door thing.' It's been with me for a very long time – years on and off – but I had convinced myself that no-one was noticing and it had slipped under the shadow of the depression and the bipolar quite nicely. I had only a split second to make a decision and I decided to tell the truth no matter how stupid it made me look – well, as little of the truth as I could get away with. They must already think me 'weird'.

"Oh, no... It's me... I just have thing about doors at the moment." Holding my breath I waited for the response, but it hadn't been enough – she asked what I meant – SHIT... so much for sweeping it under the carpet! So I explained that swing doors and wedged doors and 'back to the wall' doors were ok, but with latch type doors that needed closed, I had to shut them and then re-open and shut them again just to make sure they were working, that they would open again when I needed them to – I just HAD to – and... Well actually there was no other 'and' – no one needs to know that part. Again I paused in the hope that I could leave it there and spare us both the discomfort of further details. I really didn't have to explain any more – surely that was enough? It must have been difficult to know what to say, but then she smiled kindly and just said "Oh, right, didn't realise – that must be difficult for you." I replied that it was an ongoing thing... nothing to worry about... and the reason they perhaps were only picking up on it now was that for most of the year I got into the office first in the mornings and had the door wedged open. I secretly cursed the creeping turn in the weather; when it's colder the door gets closed and I'm stuck with this stupid little 'habit' this 'thing' that scares away unwelcome images and thoughts and makes me feel safe. It's the lesser of two evils so I live with it. Why the images and thoughts appear I just don't know. Why the playing with door handles helps I don't know. Why it comes and goes, I don't know. Where it started? – Now, I do have some ideas about that, but why my mind has taken those events and twisted them into something so rotten, I just don't know. Am I imagining an issue where none exists? I don't think so – I've watched other people – I can't see that this is normal. Is it a problem? Yes and no. The thoughts are a problem but the habit/ritual is a solution which is good, but then the solution re-enforces the link to the door and so every time I approach one it all starts again! It's all a bit 'chicken and egg'. The 'ritual/habit' itself is only a problem in that it draws unwanted attention at times and wastes so much bloody time. I've been trying to apply my new CBT skills, but so far with limited success. Is it linked to my bipolar? Apart from my ongoing anxiety issues; I don't see a direct link. Is it OCD? I think it is some form of it and it's a good job I have already decided to speak to my psychiatrist about this and the totally different but linked behaviours at work etc. Self dx is both pointless and dangerous; a proper dx wouldn't fix things but I'd feel a little better about it all. I think? I've always tried to hide this in the past.

"Understanding is precious candle light that cuts through the darkness of fear."

On my next review appointment I will try to explain some of this stuff but I'm afraid they either won't believe me or that they will be very angry that I didn't tell them sooner. I haven't been able to discuss this with anyone before – not even my Hubby – especially not my Hubby – because he is central in some of the thoughts I need to purge. Not sure how he would take that. I worry now that when I finally get the chance to sit down and talk about it, that I'll be unable to articulate my concerns or that I'll be remembering in the car park afterwards all the important stuff I should have said! – like usual!! I did try to talk about it not that long ago but I chose my timing and my words poorly and was almost immediately dismissed as fretting over stuff that was 'perfectly normal.' I've been told that I can at times have excellent insight into my condition, into my general mental health so why was I not heard? What did I do wrong? Ah well, too late now – water under the bridge – just really hoping against hope that I get a better response next attempt. To this end I have printed info from the Royal College of Psychiatrists' website and in pencil all over it scribbled all my thoughts about what it says regarding OCD. I have decided to print relevant blog entries and bring them, to bring the photos and to bring my daily notebook from work , to jot down in basic point form the main issues/rituals … all this surely will allow us to have a proper discussion. I hope. My next appointment is due just before Christmas so I won't ring in; I will wait for it to come round. Will I feel better afterwards? I don't know. This could be a mistake."

Suicidal

"Suicidal – I say one thing – they seem to hear another. Random images and thoughts of suicide visit me often but they usually hang in the shadows for only a brief moment. I rarely speak of it – I know full well that thoughts do not set me irrevocably on a path to action. These thoughts rarely scare me anymore. I live with this 'suicidal ideation' on and off but I don't loosely throw around the word 'suicidal' as to me it means so much more. These past couple of weeks though, things have been different; I found myself needing to use the 'S' word. I needed to talk about how I was feeling, what had been happening to me and to do that I had to introduce suicide into the conversation. Time has passed and for the most part I am now feeling stable, but I can't shake the disbelief and dismissal that faced me in those conversations. I felt as if my experience was being played down, as if I didn't really know what I was talking about, as if it hadn't been that serious. I had expected more. When I discuss thinking about suicide they accept what I have to say and engage in conversation but when I want to talk about actually being suicidal, suddenly it isn't real. This has all got me thinking about the word suicidal and what it means to me: because of what it seems to mean to other people, I may never raise it in conversation again. I will however share with you what I mean when I use those words. Knowing exactly where I am on this scale helps me deal better.

It breaks down into distinct stages in my thinking – there are four stages on my personal descriptive scale, each presenting a different level of risk. Professionals refer to a thing called 'suicidal ideation' but it only covers the first two on my scale as far as I'm concerned; when I use the word 'suicidal' on its own I am referring to the final two stages in general but most often the very last stage. Despite my bipolar illness, I do not use the word 'suicidal' lightly. I stupidly expected people to understand that.

1: Suicidal thinking – Quite simply finding yourself thinking about death and suicide a lot. Flashing images, random thoughts or prolonged day-dreaming, perhaps even vivid dreams. These thoughts may not always be distressing but rather quite comforting at times.

2: Suicidal planning – Finding the thought of suicide more welcoming, and considering it an ideal solution to life's presented pain and distress. You begin to linger in the arising thoughts, even inviting them so that plans can be made for the suicidal act itself. I say plans, plural, because it is not uncommon to have different plans in place concurrently.

3: Suicidal preparation – Having created a detailed plan, preparing now means gathering about you all that is necessary to carry it out. You will find yourself collecting and hiding any physical items needed, hiding them carefully until the right moment presents itself. If carrying out the plan is more imminent, you may also be doing some things such as re-arranging schedules, finding ways to say your goodbyes discreetly, putting affairs in order, giving away treasured possessions, purging computer files, shutting down social networking identities and considering the wording of a final note.

4: Suicidal – Realising that the time is right, perfectly right, and piece by piece gathering about you the physical bits and pieces you need, or placing yourself exactly where you need to be. This done, thinking yourself through the arguments for and against one last time and considering the imminent final act. Final preparations both mentally and physically for the suicide itself are all consuming. Death is invited. The final act, imminent.

You can see by the way I've broken this down that I've had years to fully consider it. I know exactly what I'm trying to say when I use any of these phrases. My obvious problem is of course that other people must have different definitions. I say one thing and they hear another. It's unfortunate."

Uneasiness I can't eat my way out of

"Like a shadow it hangs about me, intangible yet uneasiness so relentless that it fights back no matter what food I throw at it. An aero bar, two bags of crisps, a burger, three chocolate bars and a full box of Mikado chocolate sticks later, I haven't shaken it off. It was with me all day in work too but I was too busy to dwell on it: I dealt with it then by returning to old habits of self harm. My arm is tender now where I scratched the skin raw in a couple of places but that relief was unusually short-lived. I thought for sure that I could rely of my old ally, junk food, but no – looks like I can't eat my way out of this either, this, this whatever it is. I know that those little yellow pills I carry with me everywhere I go are supposed to help with stuff like this but so far I'm not noticing much of a change. Is this part of the depression? Is it the post-holiday work stress? Is it my increasing lack of sleep? Is it maybe just normal and I'm being over-analytical? Why is it so junk food resistant? I feel like something isn't right but I don't know what. I feel like something is going to happen but I don't know what. I feel a bit like I'm not even really me and I sure don't know what to think about that. Maybe it was a bit of an ask after all, to expect junk food to fix this. Perhaps there are some things beyond the power of chocolate..."

Elaine Fogarty

Random thoughts

"Am I scared of life? Scared of death? Or just scared to try? Try living? Try dying? I think I meant dying – to fail would hurt even more and to succeed would end it all. But how would I know it was over? I'd be dead. That wouldn't matter; at least I wouldn't have to live like this anymore. But what about the ones I leave behind? Not the ones that make this world unbearable but the ones who reclaim a little of it for me. What if I lose my grip? What if I get tired of clawing my way back up the cliff time after time only to be pushed off again? Each time it gets harder. My intelligence, my logic, give me tools to cope, but my heart and soul don't really want to – they are tired. Touch the fire once, get burnt, and learn to leave it alone. How many times can I be expected to reach into the flames? I'm tired. I'm scared. I don't care much about anything anymore. What's the point? What do I really want to do? How will I know it is right? Death feels right. The next morning maybe not so much... what if there is no morning? Would that be the right thing? I couldn't regret anything for I'd be dead. Or maybe I could...what happens when I die? Do I go to hell or would God understand? He'd have to for he made me; He knew I'd end up like this. Does that make it His fault or mine? Some choice isn't it... live in hell or live in hell. Thoughts spinning, jumping, jostling – too quick for my pencil to follow I want to cry but I've no tears left. What's wrong with me? Why can't I beat this? Why is it stalking me? I'm running, hiding, climbing, digging all at once – can't escape it. It's more real than anything now – I can taste it. I'm digging my nails in. I'm holding on. But I feel like someone is standing on my fingers, crushing them. It's just a matter of time. Is it? Does it have to be? No. Change the subject. Slow down. My heart feels like it's being squished, feels too much for writing...slow the thinking...slow down... find something to concentrate on... come on... think of something... RAIN... heavy rain! Watching it from inside my tent. Snuggly, warm, dry, watching it fall. Listening to the sound... and the smell and the taste afterwards. It's like it washes the world away and everything starts again fresh. Yeah, I like the rain... How did I get to rain? God, my head is so messed up!"

Change

"I know change is an unavoidable part of life and without it there can be no growth; I also know that I'd quicker crawl into a darkened room and hide than face it. Change is difficult. Learning new skills is doubly so, I'm sometimes paralysed in the face of it but I struggle on."

Diazepam, fingernails, F**k

"Intermittent car fault – months – left at dealership – diagnostic – major fault – shock – fix – £1150.02 – yes they actually charged the 2pence! – Otherwise empty credit card – damn – delivered – next day – shitty day at work – home time – SAME fault – more than once – What the hell? – Disbelief – anger – phone call – closed – message – upset – tears – chocolate binge – diazepam – fingernails – F**k – Hubby planning to camp out at their gate for opening time because I'm just too upset to deal. F**k B*ll*x F**k"

3.54am

"It's 3.54 in the morning and as usual – I can't sleep. Different thoughts tonight. I'm remembering the last time I cut myself... how it felt... wondering where would be the best place to do it again, somewhere where it wouldn't be seen. What to use? I try to think of something else and all that comes to mind is a scene from a film I once saw – where a girl deeply slashes her wrists. That's not what I need. Not tonight. I'm too tired to follow my thoughts; in fact it feels like they are racing ahead of me – somehow always bringing me back to the cutting. Gotta get these pictures out of my head. I see my thigh and wonder??? At least for a while I'd feel something different, for a while it would all go away. What would it matter anyway?"

{1/2 the A4 page is a sketch of a bare leg peeping out from under a duvet. A Stanley blade sits beside it and there are 5 question marks overdrawn in various sizes}

So obvious

"*The Matrix – The Island – The Truman Show.*
These popular films all illustrate the same idea – that we accept the reality with which we are presented. Reality isn't actually, well, um... real... it is totally reliant on perception, on the extent to which we invest in it. These films show us just how 'reality' is in fact a mere construct; they also share the theme of challenging that construct, of breaking free. What has all this got to do with me? Well, in light of my bipolar illness and my recent experiences, I can totally identify with the idea of constructed reality. My reality is a construct of my emotions and experiences – it is as real to me as yours is to you. When I cycle into depression my reality shifts seamlessly to a miserable and hopeless existence, bereft of love

and joy and hope. It is all I know. It is all that exists. It is the reality that stretches out unchallenged in front of me. Of course it's real. Everywhere I look the world is miserable and cruel, the air is filled with the stench of despair, and my only purpose is to find a way out of the torturous existence. There are no memories of better days and sounds of loved ones laughing; such things cannot even exist in this state. My reality in depression is absolute – I believe it because it is real – it is real because I believe it. I will vehemently defend my reality. In my dreams, it is the reality I am presented with. When I wake it is the reality I am presented with. Why would I challenge it? It IS real.

In *The Truman Show*, he found a door. In *The Matrix*, he took a pill. In *The Island*, he climbed a ladder. Me, I listened to a quiet anomalous whisper. Any reality is only as good as the belief that holds it together. If I begin to doubt the reality with which I am presented then it is destined to die. The reality that put me in harm's way is gone now, shattered by a new and more hopeful one. I can't help but look back and wonder how I ever allowed myself to be taken in? How could I ever have accepted that lie? It all seems so obvious now."

Aberration

"I was doing ok; my episodes had come and gone over the past year and I'd taken them for what they were and coped quite well. I've even made progress in relation to my anxiety and self-harm issues. I am genuinely proud of how well I dealt with my bipolar stuff recently. But – there it was – it wasn't so much a rollercoaster ride, but a derailment. Thing is... still don't quite know what happened this past weekend. As I was choking on dust and re-arranging and alphabetising my DVD collection this afternoon I began to figure it out. My episode of depression was melting away and I fully expected to see it gone completely within the week. I felt in control and I was glad to see that wonderful 'mellow' feeling begin to reassert itself. I had no reason to expect the crisis that whacked me like a 40ft truck. I name Hubby as my rock, my anchor, the one thing that more than anything keeps me going, gives me a REASON to keep going. I rely on him so deeply that it is engrained in my thinking, my behaviour, my hopes, plans and dreams. My identity is so tied up with him that the thought of losing him scares me stupid. Some of my OCD behaviours are tied into this fear of losing him. I just don't want to live a life that doesn't have him in it. We're close – been together 28 years and married 21 of those. He's the better part of me. I love him with everything that is in me to give – but – on Saturday night I knew I'd lost him. It may not have been real, but every fibre of my being somehow KNEW it was real – that I'd lost him. Things were said, best not repeated; each word reached through me and tore me apart from the inside. The love of my life was gone – I didn't recognise this man. The room around me began to zoom in and out around me like a 'vertigo' shot in a cartoon. All the sounds fell suddenly quiet and I knew what I had to do – I had to run, run fast and far; maybe if I ran far enough I could outrun the unbearable pain. I grabbed my bag and my keys and I got into the car and just drove – I couldn't think clearly and I couldn't fight off the dark and hopeless thoughts that rushed at me. I couldn't live without him, I thought. What did I do wrong? That's it then – there's no reason to go back, to go home, hell – no reason to live. The one small part of me that remained calm and logical tried to talk me down, to challenge the dark thoughts, to proffer some small degree of hope. I pulled in to the industrial estate and locked the doors then I sat for almost 15 minutes trying to decided whether to listen to that quiet little voice or not. I was suicidal. The more I thought about it, I realised I was in crisis and needed help, but I was so messed up I couldn't decide whether to find a hospital A&E, phone my mental health crisis team or return my Hubby's persistent mobile calls. A&E or CMHT would probably land my back on the ward (wasn't sure I wanted that, was scared I might need it). I resisted the urge to contact them because there was still a chance that a chat with Hubby would magic away the pain and magic away all the dark thoughts; I rang him. We talked, we cried, we talked and we cried and eventually I responded to his pleas to tell him where I was, to let him come get me, to come home, to let him hold me tight and hug away the pain. I took a couple of days off work because it's been a lot to get my head around and I was still very unsettled. It's intense. I go back tomorrow because I need to get back into my routine. I think that's best. Hubby and I are good, better than good – I feel safe and loved and I'm even laughing again. Such a turnaround. It's strange to me that I can be thrown into the depths of utter despair on a Saturday evening and feel as calm as I do this Tuesday afternoon. The meds were working fine, the bipolar cycles were predictable and with much less intensity or longevity; I was coping well. Saturday was an anomaly, an aberration, a reaction to perceived crisis that then became crisis: I am proud of myself for having found strength amidst all those dangerously dark moments to challenge them and look for a better path. (Thank God for CBT) I'm proud of myself for accepting that words said and words heard are not always the same thing. I'm proud of myself for emerging intact from a storm that sought to sweep me from this earth. I'm here. I'm with Hubby. I'm getting on with my life. I love my Hubby and he loves me – I don't ever want to lose sight of that again. I don't understand where that sudden swing of extremes came from but it's over now. I survived it and I'm moving on."

Lost

"I'm sat in my car, alone, with all the doors locked and I nervously watch every light, every movement about me. I'm parked up in a dimly lit access road to an industrial estate; the journey here took over an hour but as night fell, it seemed longer. I hate driving. Driving scares me and I will usually only follow a few well-tested quiet little routes – work, mum's, doctors – that kind of thing. But – things were said today, said before morning tears had even been forgiven; the details are not needed here but they lurk still in my mind. I had to walk away, to run away. I had to get out before I broke down completely. Certain things should not have to be repeated – I had no words left to explain that. I grabbed my keys and my bag and got into the car and then tried to outrun the growing despair. I needed distance... lots of distance. I've done this before – aimlessly walked the country roads on starless nights in the foulest of weather – miles, the further the better. Then, as tonight, it began as simple escapism, but soon slipped into something much more sinister – looking for a way to escape everything, permanently. When I took to wandering the streets, Hubby would usually find me and bring me home safely, but tonight I had an hour's advantage and a car; I told myself I was untouchable. The phone kept ringing but I didn't answer it. I had nothing new to say. I picked direction randomly at each junction, well – bar avoiding scary motorways: I ended up here, wherever here is. I'm lost. Genuinely and hopelessly lost, and alone, dangerously alone. I finally pulled in. It was a moment of perfect potential; tonight was the night that almost was. I finally returned Hubby's call because I became scared of the feelings, the thoughts, that were filling my mind, they were getting worse. A small part of me ached to be held by him again and be told that he loved me and that he would protect me, make it all better: that same small part of me trusted that things could get better and so I went along with it – I made the call. We talked and I know home is where I should be now, but I have no idea how I got here and even less how to find my way back. As the cold dark night ticks by me I find myself embarrassed by my predicament, but, at the time, escaping the pain was all that mattered. Everything is dumped now. The doors are locked. I begin to feel safer. Hubby is coming to get me, I hope to hug the remaining panic and despair away. I am so scared of having to trace that busy road home but I shall be so happy to curl up in my seat again; I shall be even happier as promises of better times are made new. Some things should never need repeated. Some things cry out for repetition; it gives them strength, helps them grow. Words of love sound good on the phone and in the absence of a hug, they wrap themselves around me, keeping me warm until Hubby finds me. Not long now."

Alone

"Last night, before I climbed into bed, I texted my best mate to let him know what had happened and that I was OK that I was safely back at home. He replied with a sweet message this morning asking how I was and reminding me to call him next time I needed someone to talk to, that it would have been easier and safer than doing what I did. It made me smile but I couldn't just reply with a tiny 'OK thanx'. I needed to try and explain just how complicated the whole thing can be and how, right when I really should be talking to someone, I feel as if I can't, that there is no point. It's frustrating and adds to a growing sense of isolation. I am my own worst enemy at times but I needed to try and explain that to him. Below is the message – it rambles and dances around the issue but it's the best I could do given how I am feeling this morning. It's at times like this that I truly wish I could wave a magic wand and give folk just one day in my head – just one day, and see how they hold it together. I've got excellent help at the minute; I have great meds and an impressive arsenal of coping strategies... Yet, despite all that, I still found myself sitting alone in the dark in a strange town over an hour's drive from home, with only thoughts of suicide to keep me company. – Thanx for the kind thoughts but sometimes I don't want to talk. I can't talk. That moment was passed last night. It's all very overwhelming. There was nothing 'comfortable' about my own home last night, nothing 'easy' about it. I was trying to escape, to outrun the stuff that was causing me pain. I didn't run far enough or fast enough... it all followed me. I was seriously thinking about giving up, so tired of fighting it, so tired of my life. I know things look simple to you but it's not that simple and it takes everything I have to stay on top of it all. Even if I had lifted the phone there is nothing I could have said that could have made you understand. You have an engineer's mind. If it's broken, find fault, apply repair, job done. My life doesn't work that way. The only thing 'simple' in my life is my plan for how to leave it. Most days I hardly think about it and others it's all I can think of. My good moments are higher than other people's and folk love to tag along, but my bad ones take me places no one wants to follow. I'm messed up, but at least I'm here today... Last night was a night that never happened. I didn't phone you because I didn't have the words to explain how low I was, didn't think I could handle the whole thing being over-simplified and my reality being dismissed. It's the same reason I didn't reply to Hubby's calls. I love you both, but sometimes even you can't understand, and on nights like last night I just don't have it in me to offer new explanations. You and Hubby both... Your kind words are appreciated, but they address the issue like a water bucket to a bushfire. I couldn't handle that. I'd quicker ring if I didn't have to explain the inexplicable... Or answer a million questions. Or make promises I couldn't be sure to keep. Or defend myself against judgements and assumptions. I guess what I really needed last night, all I ever really need, is the telephone equivalent of a lingering hug. I know you really care for me ... I'm sorry I didn't call last night."

Overslept

"I overslept yet I look and feel like I haven't slept at all. I look in the mirror and I'm pale with heavy red looking eyes on the verge of tears. I haven't cried yet but part of me so wants to – needs to – I alone know why. Everything feels heavy and achy. Even walking feels like a real chore. I'm slow, quiet and I feel like I'm just pretending. Yet – here I am – in work trying to convince myself I'm normal... I took two minutes to record how I felt but now I'm stuck... staring at the page, doodling, staring into space...I've no interest in actually getting some work done... but I need this job... I have to try. I've coped before, I need to try. The paperwork is under this pad but I can't seem to get to it. Can't write anymore – I really want to hedgehog, to wish the world away, but I made it into work, I owe it to them to actually get some work done... God, this is going to be a long day but I will do it somehow."

{A large ornate mirror is drawn diagonally across the page, Text crosses over it and there are various small doodles including ZZzzs and tears. It is also dated – rare.}

Blades

"Sometimes I pull one out from its hiding place and just hold it... feel it grow warm in my hand. Its sharp edge so sharp it's barely even there. And I wonder... will I ever actually use it? When? Will it feel like it did when I cut with broken glass? Will it feel like the last time I used a blade or could I cut deeper, longer? The glass I smashed in the bath was awkward and not very sharp, it was ragged, but the cuts were satisfying; I like blades better, though. I know what I would need to do to use this properly, but knowing isn't doing... anyway it's harder than most people realise and I doubt I'd have the strength. I'm thinking about cuts, it's a different thing entirely; a blade can take me to a place where none of this crap matters any more. Sometimes even holding one a while can make me feel better."

{Six life-size Stanley blades scattered across the A4 page, text overlapping in places.}

Cookie-cutter world

"Normal? – What is normality anyway? Is it really something I should be aspiring to?
I've been thinking about this a lot lately and I've decided that 'normal' is, at best, a perception of consistency or at worst, of conformity. I'll admit there is a certain degree of comfort to be had from consistency; it gives structure to life and makes everything so much easier. Conformity, on the other hand, seems less inviting. What is the point in living if we are afraid to step outside of the invisible boundaries of thought and behaviour imposed, instilled, from early childhood? Individuality is not an abomination – it is the affirmation of our true selves. Why hide it? Why fight it? Not that long ago I found myself longing for normalcy; I was fighting demons and I wanted to wish them away and then hide myself in the 'cookie-cutter world.' I craved normalcy because I had grown tired of my mood swings, my illness, and my life. I craved normalcy because I saw it as a way to hide. Today I challenge that word. Today, I understand that normalcy does not exist as a single entity – the only thing truly consistent about normalcy is the fact that it manifests differently for each person or group according to their shared experience and beliefs. What is normal for you is not normal for me – who's to say yours is better, that yours is right? What is normal in the UK is not normal in Africa, for example – who's to say which is right? We throw the word around so much but really, when people say something or someone is 'normal' all they are really saying is that they seem to conform to an accepted set of parameters, that they 'fit in' Who says we always have to fit in? Maybe we don't need to be afraid of being different. Maybe it's ok not to be normal."

Elaine Fogarty

Depression – What does it feel like?

"I wish there was a simple one word answer – I wish I could explain it – but I can't. Every attempt fails and I'm growing weary of trying. Yet here I am, once again searching for the worlds that will work – they won't though – they never do – you won't understand and it's not your fault – to be honest there are times I have trouble wrapping my own head around it. I'm not 'under the weather' or 'bad with my nerves' or 'lazy;' I can't 'pull myself together' any easier than a man with a broken leg could jump up and dance a jig! I'm ill. Depression is an illness and I need you to understand that I didn't choose this. Experience tells me you won't understand, but I've got to try anyway. The world you live in is like a dream to me. I'm in it – I may even be playing my part as far as anyone else is concerned, but it's not real. My world is a desolate and frightening version of yours. In my world I couldn't tell you what the news headlines were last night – I just don't care, and even if I did, watching that stuff makes me feel way worse. In my world the air is stale, colours are dull, family pretends there is nothing wrong and friends avoid you. In my world you can stand in a crowded room and scream at the top of your voice and no one will even turn their head. You're invisible, jostled around and carried along by everyone else. Even on the days when you know where you should be going and what you should be doing when you get there, you find yourself totally unable to do it. Numb; paralysed; so, so tired. People all around you and yet so terribly lonely... sometimes the silence can be deafening. In my world you could bleed to death without even a paper cut visible – no one will notice your life slipping away and each cruel or careless word is like salt in the wound. You want to grab someone and hold them tight but they forever slip from your grasp. When sleep finally comes the nights are filled with nightmares and the days are a struggle to even enter. Your world is beyond reach so I live in mine – forever out of step – so close and yet so far. In my world logic has different rules – it seems there must be a third option. Logic in my world dictates that if the 'normal' world is lost to you and life in its shadow is too painful then the solution is to simply leave. I don't want to leave – I want to join your world but I'm only fooling myself. No matter how hard I try it just never happens. I sneak in sometimes and pretend to be at home there, I can often fool others into believing I'm one of them – that I belong – but I don't – I can't – I never will. Pretending drains me and pretty soon I lose the will to maintain the illusion; sobbing, I limp back into the darkness and lick my wounds. Each attempt ends the same way and so pretty soon the choice is clear – it's drown slowly in despair or escape into nothingness. Feeling nothing is preferable to feeling the pain. Do I want to die? – NO – I

106

want to live – but not like this... Sometimes I get moments of perfect clarity and your world makes sense to me – I know the answers. I have perspective you will never have and it all seems so simple – life could be sooo much better, life could be worth fighting for and I know exactly how to make it all work. I know how we can all be happy... and then it hits me... just who am I going to tell? Who would listen to me? In your world my perspective doesn't matter and my answers are the ramblings of a fool. So here I sit – stuck in a world that shadows yours and faced with a stark choice – to muster my dwindling reserves one last time, or save myself the pain and simply give up... to reclaim my life just long enough to end it. So there you go – that's what depression feels like, for me, for today. Tomorrow may be totally different but right here, right now is all that matters because someone like me never really knows if there will be a tomorrow."

Hurt would live

"Words fly from the weapon with venomous purpose: they find their target and Hurt falls to the ground, dazed, confused and bleeding out. Instinctively, Anger rushes forward and shields Hurt's body with his own, but for a while at least it would seem they are safe, cover provided by the ruins of trust and dependency. Anger props her head up slightly and smiles down at her as he fastens on the bandage of the field dressing. Hurt will live, but he knows that one more serious hit like that and she'll be gone – she'll be using those open tickets and flying off – she'll be drawing about her all the elements of her carefully constructed plan – she will have grown tired of all the fighting – she will be gone. Anger knew that hurt was battle weary and had little fight left in her; he couldn't let her go. He brushed the hair back off her face and whispered an important nothing, then he launched himself around the corner and into the line of fire – the noise of weapons fire was loud, but Anger's voice boomed above it as he ran, "Leave her alone, why don't you take on someone your own size!? You want a fight? You got one!" Having by some miracle escaped the hail of fire, the upsurge of power within Anger was now violent and explosive and he spat these words out as he tackled the shooter to the ground. There followed a vicious fight; as they rolled around in the mud it became apparent that they were locked in something quite futile, they were so equally matched that little was visible but the cloud of testosterone and adrenalin. The cause of the conflict was long lost and bloodied knuckles pounded blindly until, suddenly, Hope the medic jumped from his vehicle and intervened. Anger snarled as he reluctantly backed down and then, as his breath settled and he glanced towards the hill, he knew he had done it – he'd bought Hurt enough time to escape. The image of her shadowy body disappearing into the trees made him smile. She would live. She would spend time with Love as she healed and would remind herself that a ceasefire was entirely possible. Part of her needed to be on the battlefield with her beloved Anger but deep down she knew a ceasefire would be for the greater good. In her absence, Anger returned to camp and busied himself as best he could, fighting back the distracting scent of her hair and the curl of her smile; neither knew when they would meet again and both very aware that should the ceasefire come, they would become refugees. Hurt would live – that was all he cared about. Anger isn't always the bad guy."

Done talking

"Same as last Wednesday morning, same as last Wednesday evening. I'm still choking back the disbelief... Same stuff... after what happened... what almost happened. We agreed I should feel free to talk. B*ll*x... It doesn't work. It will never work. I'm done talking... Better to suffer in silence than to speak out and suffer worse. I'm keeping things to myself from now on. I'm done talking. I learnt the hard way that it does no good. The only way I can protect myself is to trust no one, believe no one, and rely on no one. I was a fool to believe things had changed; at least I knew where I stood when I lived alone in a crowded life. I didn't escape in the car tonight. I went to bed, to wrap myself in darkness and shutdown; it's all I know to do. I can't even think right now, it hurts too much."

Icy fingers

"They tell me to be careful with excesses of caffeine and alcohol. Good advice I suppose for anyone, not just a gal like me with bipolar disorder. Something to do with trying to avoid stuff that can push the mood in one extreme or the other... I wasn't really listening – as evidenced by the rather full glass of Baileys sitting beside me now with icy fingers melting into it deliciously. Don't get me wrong now, my days of matching the men drink for drink in pubs are long gone, but until lately I was still taking a few glasses now and then. When I switched to my new anti-psychotic I found I developed a low tolerance so more or less gave up on alcohol all together. Getting drunk on one beer wasn't much fun. Tonight though, as I settled down to watch *Shawshank Redemption*, I felt the need for a little liquid comfort and creamy Baileys fitted the bill nicely. It's been a long hard day and depressed or not, I just needed a wee icy double – well maybe two, after all it's a long film."

Recurring

"Just over two hours to go in work – really don't know how the hell I am going to put two hours in... my work is very well caught up, all things considered, in fact better than many other Fridays, but I just can't focus any more. My mind is completely somewhere else and I find myself staring at the same page for twenty minutes now. Thank God it's break time. Maybe it's the approaching weekend that is making it all fresh in my mind again? I just don't know. I'd love to just go home but how can I? – Two Fridays in a row recorded as 'home early' and then the long weekend – it would be misinterpreted and I would rather not explain myself. It's not the distraction itself that bothers me, that's a common Friday occurrence for me, but it's the reason for the distraction; recurring images of what could have happened, recurring thoughts, recurring fears. This is no way to get work done. I literally can't think straight. It's going be a long two hours."

Shakespeare in Mandarin

"My seven-year-old nephew was adamant that today's first order of business was - Go to nearest town, Find participating shop, Buy the paper that has the voucher, Get FREE LEGO!!!! Now, for those of you without seven-year-old nephews, I should explain that failure to get the advertised free Lego will result in hyperventilation, floods of tears and prolonged misery for all adults involved. We got the lego and he clung tightly to that little packet as we browsed other shops. All was good in the world. It didn't last long. My other nephew pulled on my mum's arm and announced that he needed to go to the toilet: my mum has difficulty walking and so she asked me to take him to the public toilets on up the town a bit. When I said that I didn't know where to go, a total stranger started to give directions. A wave of panic began to rise inside me. It was an unfamiliar town and I wasn't at all clear on where she meant. I'm not good on my own. I'm not good in strange places. I'm not good with directions. The poor kid was really in a hurry. I took a deep breath and started to walk off with him, then Mum stopped me and started to give me directions to a better place... I'm sure her directions were spot on but I only heard broken words – the rest was a garbled recitation of Shakespeare in Mandarin. Panic was clawing its way up into my throat and I heard myself mumble something about not totally understanding the directions. The poor lad was still waiting. I felt so stupid. I felt so useless. Hubby thankfully stepped in and took him off to the toilets while all we walked on to catch up. When I saw how close the building had been I was embarrassed. I get lost easily. I get anxious easily. Add being responsible for a child in need to the mix and it starts to become a whole other animal – a beast I am obviously ill-equipped to tame. – What must the kid have thought? Oh, I am so bloody useless at times – so embarrassing. But hey, *Madagascar 3* and a gorgeous steak later, I'm starting to let it go. I tell myself tomorrow will be better."

That awful shade of neglected yellow

"I gave the book as a gift about a year ago. It was all about the dynamics of a 'bipolar' relationship; I thought it would be interesting for him, helpful even. I know there are times I'm not easy to live with. Today I found it on top of a radiator, all heat curled and beginning to turn that awful shade of neglected yellow. Not a page was creased, the spine was intact, no corner turned down or bookmark tucked carefully in place. It had not been read. I wasn't angry. I was hurt. All of a sudden I felt just as unwanted and unimportant as that book. I threw it in the bin."

Gortex skin

"I hate being lied to. Someone has just caught herself out nicely in a lie; not a big lie admittedly, but a lie nonetheless. I should perhaps be upset, but instead I find it rather amusing. I'm amused and she is totally unaware that she has let anything slip. This is a new, refreshed me today and I refuse to let stupid politics to eat away at me; a different outlook born of my CBT thinking. She has what she has and she's happy, I have what I have and I'm happy, why should one really give a shit about what the other has? What one is or isn't 'supposed' to have or 'supposed' to do is actually irrelevant – selfish as it sounds, I'm just looking out for myself these days. I have to. I don't have a 'thick skin' – mine is now Gortex – rebuffed annoyances slip away today like persistent rain; I am protected, and yet I can still breathe. I hate being lied to. Yes. I am trying to be realistic though, I understand that for many it is a protective strategy and I, of all people, should understand that need. I can see that lies are not always told in malice. I can't assume that every lie told around me is personally directed at me and I can't assume that every lie discovered is a call to arms."

The moment

"It's part of the whole 'bipolar thing' that I have depression in cycles, often very serious and intense, but the highs that cycle with them often get glossed over – almost welcome because of the energy and creativity etc that they bring. I'm about a week into a hypomanic episode now (a high) and my mind is racing; I've worked my way through more 'little projects' in this one week than in the previous two months. Even taught myself how to use PowerPoint and had fun creating a mammoth presentation. I'm organising paperwork I'd forgotten I even had. I don't want to sleep so I'm sitting up watching films and re-runs when I should be in bed. I'm really distracted and can't concentrate at all. I don't care. Unfortunately, even though it happens every time and I should be prepared for it, I still find myself spending money recklessly – I try to be careful, but ultimately I fail. After all, I do have Amazon, eBay, and Argos all on browser tabs; I am addicted to online shopping.

"Hypomania is like surfing – you know eventually you're going to crash but while you find yourself up there, you may as well ride the wave and enjoy yourself!"

Because I'm being caught up in the whole hypomania thing and my mind is all over the place and just never stops, I am consciously trying to find ways to calm myself a little. I've been listening to a lot of relaxing music like classical and Enya and that is nice – especially in work where I sit working away with the earphones running from the phone on the desk. I have a background in yoga, meditation and relaxation techniques but often find it difficult to access these skills when I need them. When the world around me gets busy or indeed, as now, when my own mind is overactive, it's so nice to just read through this poem and be reminded of an important truth – all there really is, is the moment."

{Full text of my own poem 'This Moment' – see poetry section.}

18½ hours

"Cup of coffee in hand I sit watching *Star Trek* and the evening stretches out in front of me. It's 5.45pm and all is well – I feel good – I feel better than good – I feel great. So, what's unusual? – I'm just out of bed! A couple of days ago I became aware that the hypomania that had enveloped me for almost three weeks was finally easing. My energy levels began to level out, I was eating

more normally and I lost the urge to be doing twenty things at once; strangely, I was ok with that. Normally I would have fought to defend my hypomania, but I knew in my heart that it was time to let it go. For the next couple of days all seemed quite normal except for a predatory tiredness that refused to leave me as my system readjusted. Last night I went to bed around 10pm as usual. I woke with my morning alarm as usual too but it did me no good – I instantly knew that there was no way I could function at work – I wasn't even sure I could get out of bed, let alone drive a car safely and then sit juggling papers and updating data. I certainly didn't want be around people; I wanted to be alone, asleep, and very very alone. I made the call to the answer machine at work and, having excused myself for the day, drifted back into a welcome and effortless sleep. All together I slept 18 ½ hours last night – 18 ½ hours – a 'crash' that fully lived up to its name. I woke up and it was gone; the hypomania had run its course and I was a different me. I plan to go into work again tomorrow and because it's a Friday and the last day of the week, it will be a good test of just how things have settled. During these past three weeks hardly anyone in work noticed there was a change in me – really, I can't blame them, after all I was much more productive, much more sociable. I was working well and getting lots done – just what I am supposed to do. Because I lied when asked, no one realised that I was barely eating and I certainly wasn't going to volunteer the fact that I was only sleeping 2-3 hours a night or that my bank balance and credit card had both taken heavy damage. They all know I have bipolar disorder but they rarely pick up on my difficulties linked to hypomania, they would easier pick up on the symptoms of depression. This is totally understandable.
I rode the wave until it crashed and now my life picks up again and I get on with things; I get back to normal – whatever normal is."

Hypocrite's way out

"I was just settling in for a nap... there were voices coming from one of the other bays but I only caught enough to recognise that someone was feeling really vulnerable + scared. She kept talking about suicide + how the voices were getting louder – pushing her. She got upset and walked out of the room. What happened next REALLY upset me. She was barely out of the room when I heard a voice say, "I shouldn't have to listen to that. People going on and on about killing themselves – it's the hypocrite's way out anyway – so selfish." I was sitting there thinking about how I was struggling myself. I'm told I should talk about it, but what's the point if that's the reaction you get? I don't know how to feel now! She didn't know what she was talking about anyway, because it's not the hypocrite's way out – it's simply the only way out. I don't know whose voice that was behind the curtain but I hope to God it wasn't one of the nurses! I thought I would benefit from being on the ward, but now I'm really distressed; I don't know who I can trust. I wish I'd never agreed to come in. No – this is silly – I'm just getting anxious. I can't let this drag me down when I've been doing so well these past couple of days."

Poetry

"Yesterday was a rotten day and I can't shake it from me – it clings to my skin, seeps into my veins and labours every breath I take. I can't find the words for how hurt and unloved I feel. This, I know, will not pass easily. After a night of fitful sleep and agitation I find myself sitting downstairs much too early on a Sunday morning. My head aches and I feel nauseous; I don't want to face the day. I wish I could cry but the damn meds stole my tears months ago. Instead, I turned to drafts of poetry started long ago, but stalled mid flow. I was drawn to one in particular, and have now completed it."

Sleep

"My eyes are heavy, stinging and trying to push out the back of my head. My head is pounding and my stomach churns as if I've eaten week old prawns. I'm full of wind and feeling very uncomfortable; every muscle aches with a heaviness that I can't describe. I can catch myself clenching my teeth or biting my nails, but by now this is completely normal. I haven't slept and the memory of nightmares lingers still. I'd cry but I've no tears left – the only thing I want to do is sleep. I close my eyes and my mind jumps into a flurry of activity – random, totally unconnected thoughts – a swirl of busyness and confusion. But now there's a lap to rest my head on, there's an arm that holds me close. Slowly, very slowly, sleep comes. It's getting harder to function. I'm so tired and I'm running out of ways to explain. My dreams were always vivid, even as a child. If I rolled over quick enough I could even sometimes fall back into a version of the same dream. It's a blessing and a curse. Right now that imagination, that creativity, makes the nightmares vivid. It creates the things I fear, the things that in my pain I sometimes wish for. It makes them REAL. ⅓ of a life is spent in a dream world – it is as real as the waking world. Can one inform the other? Which is stronger – my dream self or my waking self?"

{Four neat rectangles of clear, written text, positioned at angles over the A4 page with geometric precision. No sketches or doodles.}

None of this is insurmountable

"Well, I've had a shower and washed my hair and got my jammies on. I'm sitting warm and comfy in front of the telly, relaxing, kicking back. I'm feeling strangely calm now. I'm thinking kinda clear. The fogginess of the depression has long passed now and the oscillating resignation and self doubt of this past 10 days are reconciled. Earlier today I sat in work dreaming about how nice it would be to be normal, well, by that I think I meant 'stable' and as I sit here now, I feel pretty damn stable. After all, stable isn't the absence of emotion, of moods, it's the absence of those awful irrational extremes. So I haven't been sleeping great... so I have been cutting again... so I've still got all that OCD stuff... so I've been very distracted... so I've been doing some serious comfort eating... so what? Really – none of this is insurmountable. Everyone has problems, issues, and challenges – I wanted normal – guess I found it – or it found me. Perhaps I've slipped through the looking glass so many times I can't recognise normal any more. I really don't know, but tomorrow might just be ok."

The hand

{A composite doodle on A4 paper done in shaded pencil. The main shape is a large circle, perfect but for the fact it has been drawn with a portion cut off by the right page edge. Over that there is a clear life-size left hand with a heavy outline as dark as the circle's. At the bottom of the circle there is a cluster of doodle images – a campfire, a heart, and one of those pendants designed to break the circle in two so that each half can be worn by a different person. Where the wrist meets the outline of the circle there is rope across half of it with a sizeable knot and trailing ends. The other half of the wrist sits next to a darkly shaded poinsettia flower; about it, two realistically shaded full size blades (one dripping with blood) Below the flower, at the very bottom of the page, are two dual-colour medication capsules. To the left of the flower, in the extreme left corner, there is a softly shaded thought bubble containing the number 42 and a question mark crosses it edge. Above the blades there are two extremely dark tears and the symbol for infinity. Behind that, a brilliant sun begins to peep from the left side of the circle – only half of it is visible. About this there is a small clock face smiling at ten to two; there is a band/belt of some kind around it in much the same way the rings hang around Saturn. There is an implication of movement backed up by two arrows on the circle's edge – one pointing clockwise, the other anticlockwise. Finally, the words 'Reaching out' and 'Slipping back' are marked out in very heavy lower case with question marks – one to the top of the drawing and one to the bottom.}

Floating

"Lately I've felt like I've been floating on the surface of life, just drifting, doing nothing, going nowhere. The days blur into each other and they all seem the same to me. I don't watch the news or engage in office chit-chat; the world could be scheduled for destruction tomorrow and I'd have no clue. What's worse, I don't even think I'd care. Thing is – these past few days, I've begun to feel a current rise up beneath me; its pulling me gently and I'm having to swim against it just to stay in one place. I don't like this feeling – it's disturbing."

Side-swiped

"Just when I was almost getting to grips with my current episode of depression, I get totally side-swiped by a nauseating wave of anxiety; literally nauseating. I haven't felt at all well all day and now as I try to settle for sleep it rushes up inside me. Through this depression so far I've managed to work all but one day (which is great) but after last week's lovely holiday I'm now stressed about going back. Everything on my desk will be all crooked or in the wrong place? The papers in the trays won't be cornered? They should all be on the left and I know I'm the only one who cares about that... but still. My filing might be disturbed? There will be a big workload in my in tray? The stuff others have done with best intentions will shout at me until I retrace it all. Even though that work is always done and done right, I stress. I'll be compelled to recheck it through all my stages again. I'll know it's unnecessary, but I'll HAVE to do it. That will take more time and I'll be playing catch-up for still longer. I'm my own worst enemy I know, but I just can't help it. Damn OCD. And what about my spreadsheets? Oh, I know, I can hear myself... What's the big deal you say? ... For God's sake – what an ungrateful b*tch, folk are trying to help, the work needs done and that's that! Get over yourself! I know. I know. But then I also know what will be waiting for me when I go in. I know I'll have to choke back the overwhelm and rising frustration and smiling, discuss the relaxing holiday I wish I'd never taken. I hate first days back and tonight the anticipation is making me physically ill. My head is pounding. I feel my throat closing in, which is probably just as well for I feel like I may be sick at any moment. I'm fed up climbing the stairs to the bathroom and on top of it all I can't quite calm my breathing. It's unsettling and as I knew I wouldn't sleep I've stayed up way too late and started this to try and get it out of my system. I can hardly see this phone straight. I can hardly think straight. I'm a mess – and all over stuff that to others must seem trivial or imagined. I can't explain it. I can't change it. The anxiety meds didn't work earlier so I'm going to resort to my sleep meds to try and ease this horrid feeling and perhaps let me get some rest. I may be too wound up for that to even work but I've got to try because this anxiety doesn't mix well with depression. I so want to just curl up and wish the world away – sometimes I just can't handle it.

Addendum
"I have been through some terrible things in my life, some of which actually happened."
Mark Twain – US humorist and author (1835 – 1910)

As often happens, the anxiety over-estimated the distress of the events to come. Things were not as bad as I'd dreaded and work completed on my behalf was of course correctly done and returned in neat ordered bundles or clipped and left tidily on the desk – a desk, I may add, that was virtually untouched apart from the hole punch sitting in totally the wrong place and gloating over its downturned angle. I can see now how pointless all that stress was. My OCD self is coping. I find myself able to adjust a lot better than I'd thought. Still feeling anxious and unsettled and a little ill but hopefully it will only take a couple of days to re-establish my routine and work through all the outstanding stuff. This is all down to me, I know it, but there are ways things need to be, NEED TO BE, and until I feel they are once again right, I can't settle – I feel a little like a temp sitting at my own desk. Why the hell can't I just be like everyone else? – Why does my world have to suffer such confusion between trivialities and imperatives? I just know that that is how it is – I know it's the OCD and I accept it because, I suspect at times, it is the glue that holds me together."

Monday

"I made it to another Monday. I'm sitting at my desk with a pounding headache and eyes that just won't stay open. I'm so tired. Last night, again, I used a sleeping tablet just so I could get past the onslaught – head to pillow usually signals a free-for-all amongst the thoughts in my head; they appear from nowhere and persist most of the night – jostling for attention. The sleeping tablet at least allows me to get some rest but it doesn't always banish the darkest of dreams. It's in the quietness of night that my mind strays furthest from the path, drifts into areas I work hard to avoid during the day.

In my dreams I play out scenarios of death, of suicide. In those quiet grey hours my mind lobbies for the inevitable and even if the detail is lost upon waking, the sensations remain; despair and helplessness hang in the air, wearing me down. Today, like most before it, I had to really struggle to get out of bed, to force myself into a new day. Today, like many before it, I had to call on every bit of strength I had just to wash, dress and make it into work. I'm sitting here now because of a huge effort, wishing my lunch break could last forever – I'm here because I hope I can make it through the day somehow and maintain the illusion. That's rubbish of course! I really need some help, someone to talk to, actually – just someone to sit with me and share the silence. I've learnt the hard way though that it rarely works out that way. I should be able to tell people I'm ill but I worry that they will immediately begin to treat me differently – innocently but, still – that would isolate me even more. Dare I risk it? I've got friends here. Have I got the words? I really need take some time out to try and find myself again, to remind myself of what's good in life, an yet I can't; even a few days off work without pay will create money worries that will push further down. I'm trapped. I wish I could do flexi hours; they have no idea how much I have to struggle at times to keep the work up to date. I'm doing the work, I'm staying on top of it, I'm doing well, but it's killing me right now... I can't maintain this for much longer – I'm in too bad a place. I'm embarrassed to ask for help – don't want to create problems for everyone. I get home and I collapse, I've literally no energy left and quite often I just sit and cry. I feel trapped and helpless. The whole cycle repeats and repeats and I just get worn down. I've been here before – I know where this is heading. I'm digging my heels in and trying to fight it but it's still happening. I'm gonna snap. That scares me."

{This was written before I made the decision to be open about my illness.}

Little boxes

"I compartmentalize. Fleeting thoughts of suicide that still visit daily must not be allowed to touch the rest of my life. If they must come, I choose to deny them fertile ground in which to grow: if they must be

forever a part of me, I choose to acknowledge them and allow them to pass into that place where they can do no harm. For as long as I can, I will choose life. To someone who has never been there, never found themselves planning suicide, it must be difficult to understand what I'm trying to say. My experience of depression and suicidal thinking over the years is unique and very personal. I cannot share details because I do not wish to trigger the vulnerable and conflicted. As I sit here this evening, I do not consider myself suicidal. My personal definition of that would be to be actively planning the act, the very minutia of it, with definite and considered intent, secretly gathering around me all that was needed to carry it through. In the days and weeks running up to the suicidal stage there is a lot of what the professionals call suicidal ideation – just a way of saying 'thinking about it'. This suicidal ideation can be a precursor to actually being suicidal or, while still vague and without actual intent, can stand alone as a challenge to those stressed or in emotional difficulty – without ever leading to a more serious state. Although I have often been plagued by dark thoughts, this is not where I am today. Having experienced all these states with varying frequency and intensity since my early teens, I know it's a big step from thinking about it a lot to actively planning that one specific and final act. I received my diagnosis of bipolar disorder late in 2006, many years after having lived with the related issues and struggled with depression and the spectre of suicidal thinking. Since then, the medication has really helped to take the edge off, but I still have difficult episodes to deal with. Thankfully, since my diagnosis, I have largely been spared the despair and desperation that comes with being suicidal, and I do not find myself constantly pre-occupied with suicidal ideation. Suicide is still with me though; I doubt it will ever really leave me. Every day, every single day, even on those wonderfully full and happy ones, it jumps into my mind in some way. Usually, seconds, brief and fleeting, these images are conjured from somewhere deep inside me and I can't control them. Given my history, they are undeniable parts of me, thoughts and experiences that can't be unthought or undone. A plan, for example, once made, can never be unmade. I gave up fighting them and took a different approach. I believe I have now found a way to live with them by learning to compartmentalize. They come, but most days they don't scare me – most days I simply allow myself to see them, to acknowledge them and then I allow them to pass into that special place deep inside where they can do no more harm. When they do scare me I have learnt to actively challenge them, to negate their influence. I have become better at this since my cognitive behaviour therapy. Once I challenge the intruding thought or image it slips away just like the others.
I am aware that this strategy may not always work and that the dark

118

images and thoughts may one day begin to linger and spread insidiously until my carefully structured defences begin to fail. I am realistic but I cannot really live my life if I think too much about that – So I compartmentalize. I try to live for the moment because that's where I am now at my strongest, that's where I've learnt how to survive. I know that to compartmentalize like this is to indulge in some degree of dissociation but I still argue that it is necessary... for me... it works."

Insight

"Insight they call it – Well, what good is insight if it comes 12 hours too late? Knowing what was happening back then doesn't change the fact it was all real at the time – in every way that mattered. My mind, my body, and every sense – they all told me it was real so it was!! I lay awake for hours, fighting sleep, scared to sleep, because I knew that when I woke up, Colin would be dead! Next morning, having eventually succumb to weariness and slept, I woke to find Colin alive and well and I was beyond relieved. The next night I should have known better – but – it happened again; I knew without shadow of doubt that if I slept, he'd be dead when I woke again. It was incredibly distressing. I watched him sleep and I sobbed quietly as I whispered goodbye. It was real. Where was my insight then? I could have done with some – I could have been saved from all that pain. Now I feel a residual confusion, as if caught between two clashing realities. NOW my insight shows up and explains that the mind loves to play tricks. I feel embarrassed. I feel angry. I feel scared – yea actually, mainly scared."

Been there

" 'I've been there, I've tried and failed, and even I can't say that I know how you feel. Yes, depression has been part of my life, yes I did try to kill myself – but I can't tell you what to do. I can't tell you anything except that I care – I'll listen if you need to talk and I'll give you space if you need it. All I ask of you is a promise – that you'll call if it ever gets too much – me, anyone, but that you won't do anything until you make the call. Only you know where the line is; if you feel the urge to cross it you should call first – Please. Just promise me that.' A quiet, subtle nod and then a hug. No lecture, no judgement, not pressure. Just the feeling that maybe, just maybe, I wasn't alone. That night I actually slept."

Buns

"I got 2½ hours sleep last night... I sat up really late, well, technically, really early. When I did do to bed I slept for what seemed like 5 minutes and then I found myself in the kitchen making buns! It was still dark outside and I was baking – I knew what was happening – I knew it was the hypomania – somehow it felt ok. After the buns came out of the oven I sat down at the computer and ran through all the questions on my latest correspondence course module; I answered the whole paper."

I am raining

"I am raining – What a strange thing to find myself thinking... were my thoughts just a bit scrambled this morning or is there some other explanation? If I disregard the physical body for a moment and recognise the true self, neither mind nor body, but the source of both, then I understand my experience as part of a greater whole. Quite literally, my true self is part of the universal whole and as such, there is shared experience, shared action, shared existence and shared responsibility. This would extend to all the elements in nature. My thought, "I am raining," could have been a brief realisation of this truth – a fleeting communion with all that exists, an immersion in the ultimate truth. On the other hand, and quite worryingly, perhaps there is the possibility that this thought crept into my mind because, subconsciously I believed I had the power to MAKE it rain. Me, Elaine, the flesh-and-blood Elaine... On some level the rain had started because I willed it so. I want to believe the first one. That would be welcome. I'd rather realise a higher spiritual awareness than find myself delusional. That said – there's a part of me that points to the more obvious explanation – I am simply living with an incoherent mind and quite literally, can't think straight. I know what I would choose to believe."

Conversation

"Working through and keeping up appearances – it all takes a huge amount of energy and that's something I'm already sadly lacking. The effort involved in just one hour of polite conversation and socialising is immense – I really don't know where I am going to find the reserves. All the while I'll be scrambling inside, hoping to escape the cheerful chatter and find somewhere dark and quiet. It's gonna be tough, but on goes the smile and off I go."

Blood dreams

"4.54am. Fell asleep but it didn't last long. Really bad dream...
Blood, Lots of blood. Mine – I think – but I never saw myself, only
the blood. Pools of gloopy, thick, dark red and splashes of finer
stuff. Can't remember how – or why – or as I said, even who – but it
must have been me. Me, and yet I was just standing there looking
at it... Like looking at myself I guess. Weird. I've just spent 10
minutes trying to calm down and have only just realised the 'itch'
that I'd been rubbing was the scar from the last cut. A tiny, healing
scar, so fine it looks almost like a cat scratch; the blade had been
fine and sharp. Somehow I needed to touch it, to check it was
closed, that it was healing. Actual suicide dreams are easier to deal
with -
I don't like these ones where I just see blood."

{Shaded sketches of three large pools of blood.}

Normal

"I wish someone could explain to me just what 'normal' means, but
of course no one can because it's relative. Your normal, my normal
– different. My mood swings are normal for me and for many years,
I thought everyone else was the same. So I've decided to stop
using the word – it is pointless because it can never hold any
meaning. Instead when I find myself in that rarest of places, a
space between episodes, I say that I am 'stable.' Yes, it's evasive
but I just can't wrap my head around what 'normal' is supposed to
me for me."

Sorry for myself

"I'm feeling very sorry for myself – trying to lose weight – had lost
about 7lb, but it's back on. I'm so disheartened – feel like just giving
up. My self esteem is in the gutter and, largely due to my new
meds, I'm 4 stone overweight. Is it worth it?"

Pendulum

"The pendulum is swinging. I can feel it. Today I'm very down –
generally low and irritable. This is how the depression sometimes
sneaks up on me. I need to be careful."

Even

"Is it just a matter of perception? It must be. Should I mourn the familiar rollercoaster as I sit here in this drifting log flume? I asked for help and I got it but now I just feel so flat; I've only ever known the extremes and I'm finding it hard to adjust. Should I be happy that the meds have introduced this new landscape? Is normal life meant to be dull and flat or does it just seem that way to me because I am ill-accustomed? I feel like part of me is slipping away forever and I don't really know what to think about that. Well, they do say 'be careful what you wish for' I guess it is all about perception and when I hang out in their world a while, I'll start to see things their way, become one of them, become normal. Change and growth are part of life so I'll just have to stick around a while and see what happens."

Email at work

To: Elaine
Hi Elaine – I'm very conscious that I haven't been able to catch up with you lately – I don't want you to think that I have abandoned you – your email mentioned a dip in mood – how are you finding things at the moment?

From: Elaine
Thanks – I could just say 'Not, bad thanks' as it's pretty much my standard reply when I want to acknowledge people's concern whilst holding back the details we both know they don't really want to hear. But I said I'd be totally open with you, so, since you asked... To be honest I'm only a couple of weeks in and I'm already finding things pretty tough. This one is going to be a particularly pernicious episode – I can tell – it's not coming at me directly this time but attacking from beneath, undermining all the coping strategies I've been so careful to put in place. It's a bit like trying to fend off hungry wolves with a flame and knowing pretty soon it will flicker out completely and you'll be alone in the darkness and vulnerable. Of course, as I'm up to date with all my meds, the edge will be significantly taken off and I take some comfort in knowing it's highly unlikely all these rotten thoughts will coalesce into a serious suicidal state. That's a plus at least. I've got used to the distinction over the years between thinking/planning/preparing/doing. It's easier to deal with things when I know where I am on the scale – I can adapt my strategies to suit.

Depression underlies my whole day at the minute, like a faint music soundtrack, and it's a struggle not to get too distracted, but most of the time I can still work through quite well. I can mask my feelings with smiles and chat; I can retreat in an acceptable way like breaktime walks, slipping off for meditation or just sticking in the earphones and listening to some opera – I do what I have to do and get the work done (hopefully without translating my difficulties into any kind of issue that will ruin someone else's day). While I can still do that I know I'm reasonably OK. Tuesday was the exception. I was off on Tuesday as much for everyone else's benefit as my own. Bad days happen; I'm used to that. B has been looking out for me, but so far I'm staying on top of things here at my desk and although I am definitely working slower, I'm still getting it done. When I get home and there is no workload and no need for social niceties I do tend to fall back into myself a good bit more and the thoughts that I spent all day trying to suppress come percolating up. It's never easy.

But I do what I can. So, that's where I am at the minute. "Not bad, thanks." ...Elaine

To: Elaine

I'm grateful you think you can tell me the truth of the matter – I can't begin to understand but can sympathise and you know we will all help in any way we can as far as work is concerned – keep me updated – don't think you have to struggle on alone."

{I'm fully aware of how lucky I am to be supported at work; some disclose their illness and face all kinds of problems – everyone here now knows about my illness and I don't feel at all bad about asking for help if I need it. I function well here. I have a future here. Openness has worked for me.}

Just saying

"Thumping headache... So when we pulled in to buy ice cream, I picked up some paracetamol. Hubby uses paracetamol and it's about the only painkiller I can use, thanks to my other lovely meds. We use it quite often and it REALLY bugs me that they limit purchases to small amounts. I know why they do it. I know why they think it's a good idea. I know why they think it would work. But, I know what I'm talking about here – If I found myself needing large amounts of paracetamol for, well, you know what for, no piddling small purchase policy would put me off my notion. There are options. It wouldn't work. Despite its good intentions, I really don't see how this policy stands to achieve much – it irritates me. Just saying..."

Confidence issues

"I was asked by someone very close to me to read and critique a comedy script proposal featuring a coming together of many of my favourite fictional characters. He knew I wasn't feeling well, but he also quite rightly understood I was more than happy to give it a go. I found it extremely difficult, though, not just because of my lack of concentration but, remarkably, a diminishing level of confidence. As I read it and began to mentally highlight areas of interest I found that I was doubting myself, double-guessing and over-thinking what I'd planned to comment. It made the whole thing really difficult to do and I returned it still feeling a bit uncomfortable. Had I said too much? Had I made glaring errors of omission? Could I actually be confident in the facts I had referred to? Well, it's too late now – it's away. I am still a little unsettled by my failing confidence in a subject I was previously known to be well versed in. In the past something like this would have been easy and pleasurable to do. It would be easy then to blame the current depression. I'd like to. I'm just a little worried that it's an emerging of one of those vague bipolar issues that hang around even in between mood episodes. My general confidence is already low but it is a little distressing to feel the cancer eat into areas previously left untouched

Thursday

"Today is Thursday – and it's been a good day. Not an over-the-top good day – just a good day. I'd almost begun to forget what they felt like. Folk in here have been great – staff and other patients – it's been a good space for me."

Labels

"Yet another label? But maybe this one is right? Right label might = right treatment. I'm not after a magic fix, don't even care if it's a shit load of tablets I need, I just need to finally get some balance. I had, up to a point when I was teaching the yoga but now I can't even bring myself to personal practice @ the moment. Manic depression? Bipolar II? What is it? I'd research it but I'm too tired right now. It's either buzz buzz and hardly feel like sleeping, or sleep and doze at every opportunity lately. I'm p*ssed off by all these extremes. What the hell is wrong with me? What does bipolar mean anyway? I really don't care what label I have – I just want to know how to deal – I want to get back to that place where I was able to stay on top of things, or at least tread water long enough to get more help. I hate feeling lost and out of control – with stuff like thing at least. I do feel a little bit better because for the first time, I got to talk without a vacant stare or judgemental comments. Wonder if I can really trust this guy?"

{A drawing to the top of the page of a manila label, on it the words 'Bipolar/Manic depression' Besides, it a thought bubble with the words 'Need to find out more.'}

The book

"Feeling very low at the minute – really struggling with dark thoughts. I was tidying the bookcase and lifted a fallen book to fix it – I glanced at the title – '1000 places to visit before you die'!!!!!! Is someone up there messing with me? How to totally make me feel crap!"

Wide awake and weary

"Wide awake and weary...it's a strange juxtaposition...yet at 4.41 this morning it's where I find myself. I'm scared to try going back to sleep because of the dreams that live there and I'm reluctant to actually get up, to commit to a fresh early start because I'm afraid tiredness, like some ghoulish prankster, will set upon me just as I begin to find my stride. To my reckoning I've had three hours, 15 minutes or so of sleep. Is that enough? Hey, that's close to pi, very close to pi: I'm seeing coincidences everywhere lately and feel compelled to assign them meaning; it's the death rattle of a mind that desperately needs to shut down. So, what to do? I'm too unsettled to read and can't put the TV on downstairs without waking Hubby. Guess I'm yet again stuck with lying in bed for hours just allowing the depression to think itself out. Thinking does not necessarily imply structure or logic – in fact, in times like this the picture of my mind resembles that famous image with all the stairways merging from different perspectives – it is obvious they are connected, functional, yet it is simultaneously obvious that they cannot be. It really sucks to find yourself the thoughts rather than the thinker."

Random

"I've written and destroyed more notes, poetry, journals etc than most people have perhaps written – and here I am – still writing, scribbling gibberish and insight in one mess of paper. Some stuff has gone and those that are left are rarely dated; dates are irrelevant. I'm still writing. I wonder why – I mean, I know why I write – its expression, release, even at times a compulsion. It is what it is. I mean why try to keep them. Especially now. I've shown one or two selected pages to my GP and a couple to close friends, but it isn't really for other people – it's just for me. I read them back sometimes and even I don't understand them – so why bother then? Will I ever share them? – Doubtful. I've been told to bring my notes to the ward when I'm admitted. They seem to think it's a good idea. I'm tempted not to. I'm tempted to 'edit' down the pile. I don't know if I am ready for other strangers to be reading my most personal stuff. I feel vulnerable, perhaps even ashamed: sharing these notes could do more harm than good. I'm scared to share. Lately I've been frightened by how easily the other part of me wants to give in, by how close I have come yet again to ending it all. I'm frightened I may lose control; my notes are the glue that holds me together, they keep me grounded. Guess I'll keep them after all."

Day release

"Oddly enough I feel like writing a little slower and a little more legibly tonight. So how did my day go? Out about 9.30am immediately after meds + getting dressed and changed. Dad picked me up and we headed to theirs for some brekkie. It was lovely to be round the table with family again. My sister arrived and the kids just went into overdrive, so excited to see me. I felt pulled in ten different directions at once – I loved playing with them but it all became a bit overwhelming. And the noise – oh the noise. I'd hoped for an easier afternoon but we ended up in a shopping centre – not ideal, but I coped quite well. I had a phone call from my best mate too, which was really great. When Hubby picked me up, it was round to my in-laws for tea and from there back to the ward. I'm glad I did it but I hadn't expected it to take so much out of me – I'm exhausted. I need to relearn how to be sociable."

The colours of my mind

"The greyness still hangs about me this morning like a faint watermark above the blue, laying claim to my life; I am aware of it but also fully aware that it is gradually fading , melting into a welcome mellow green. It has been a difficult few weeks but at least my meds and support held ground against the assault of dangerous and disturbing black; in old battles best forgotten, black had pushed through meagre defences and shrouded my life with a suffocating purpose, a longing for death. But not this time. Not today. While I yet carry soft blue, there is green on the horizon, my precious green, my refuge against the storms of bipolar and its allies, my green first born of meditation and mindfulness but now increasingly spontaneous, my green – my balm on battle scars. The canvas of my life was once dominated by broad strokes of grey and yellow, indeed of stronger Black and Orange, of intense and crippling browns. In the past I swept the brush easily over Navy that repeatedly tried to assert itself despite my attempts to wish it out of existence. My bipolar self has always painted in broad strokes and strong colours, portraying at best, a world of crimson and purple in contrast to yellow and red, and at worst, the violent and rapidly cycling extremes of black and white. Lately though, I have rediscovered the greenness of life and I can begin to unleash my silver and allow lemons to flourish.

I know that I no longer have to view the world from behind my cream veil or accept the limitations of alluring peach: I am more than the palette of my colours and, with all the pink and rose I am lucky enough to enjoy, I can create a canvas that speaks to my precious hard won gold, tempered by a subtle white."

Shut up

"Shut up!! I cried for an hour for no good reason. I took back control. I left you all behind for a while and headed to the beach in meditation. I felt better – positive – hopeful. Even got to sleep early, about 12. Now it's 3.20am + I'm wide awake with you in my head again. Why is it always you @ night? I don't want you – go away – your whispers seem louder at night. I don't want to think about suicide. I don't want to dwell on how alone I am. I don't want to dwell on how no one seems to give a shit if I live or die. I can't even think past tonight. I don't want to think and plan – I don't want your pictures either – P*ss off. Go away! I hear myself thinking it, but I know it's you. I made that decision – remember! I don't want that! Stop filling my head with all the reasons it would be better to die. Go away. What if you're right? I don't care if you're right. F**k off!

It's a trick – you can't be right – I'm just not listening – LaLa LaLa, LaLa, LaLa, LaLa – not listening – get out of my head! Leave me alone. I've got enough to deal with without fighting you. You had your chance and you blew it – now b*gger off back into the shadows. Leave me alone! Not doing it, not planning it, not thinking about it tonight. Clear off and take those pictures with you – blood, blades, pills and more – let it go – let me sleep."

{The top of the page has a speech bubble filled with expletives}

Can't find the words

"Came home from work today at about 11am. I just couldn't function; every piece of paper I lifted, everything I went to do seemed too complicated, too difficult. Polite conversation was beyond me. I just couldn't concentrate – my head was all over the place, edgy and totally distracted with a sudden upsurge in negativity and self pity. I've had days like these before and I know it is best to take a step back rather than force on and end up making things worse. I worry that my time at home here will be misunderstood Given that it is Friday, some may feel I simply wanted a nice long weekend. I remind myself that they do understand. I can't do anything about the feeling so I choose not to think about it. Some time has passed but as I sit here at tea time, I really don't feel any better. I thought to update my blog but find I have nothing to say. I can't find the words to fully describe things – simply put – I feel crap and I can't function. I'd love to cry, but the meds have stolen my tears."

Longing for normality

"Last night, strange and troublesome thoughts kept me awake. I sat up two extra hours vaguely watching documentaries about penguins and ice flows, but my mind stubbornly refused to switch gear. The choice was simple… toss and turn all night like a demented tossy turny thing, or take one of those sleeping tablets that would claim the first couple of waking hours as sacrifice (they work a little too well sometimes). Meds it was. I slept. My waking self struggled to come to terms with the new day but I made it – it's now 5pm – half an hour to go and I can tick off another day survived. Don't get me wrong, I know everyone has trouble getting up from time to time, has difficulty dragging themselves through a difficult day, but I am ill equipped to deal with normality right now – I'm still stuck in that abnormal repeating loop of what recently happened and what might recently have happened – it's hard to think about anything else. I am spent. Hubby and I are going round to my parents' house this evening and I'm hoping my little nephew will be there still; he had to have an emergency operation last night but is home now. I rang him earlier but I want to see him. I'll have to wear my fleece when I call because the cuts on my arm are really prominent and I've always tried to avoid that conversation with the kids – tonight is definitely not the right time – there are more important things to talk about. Spending time with family will do me good, even if it's only for a short while. That's normal. I'm hoping that if I keep doing 'normal' stuff, I'll gradually begin to feel 'normal' again and these persistent thoughts will fade into memory and allow me a few months stability. I haven't had a 'stable' Christmas in a couple of years; it would be so nice to greet the season with a smile. When depressed these past three years I hadn't even put up a tree. Last year the cards just sat in a pile on the table. Perhaps this year I can put up a tree and play music and enjoy the whole Christmas thing – that would be sort of normal – that would be so good."

What are the odds?

"I'm not good with mathematics – just what are the odds of the same girl getting accidentally locked in a room TWICE in ten years?? First time I was a ball of energy and was seriously into my spring cleaning. I had attacked a tiny little store which we all referred to as 'the hell hole' that gives you an idea of the state of this glorified cupboard. It was in the back of the showroom, off the beaten track. There was no light inside because it was barely a room after all, and as a large cupboard, the door could only be opened from the outside and so had to be wedged open when in there looking for stuff. So there I was that afternoon, door wedged as I carried filled bin bags out and shifted computer monitors and other assorted crap. All was ok until I caught the wedge with my foot and heard the door slam behind me. I hammered the door and kicked the door to the point of putting a huge hole in it, but I couldn't get it open. Stood there in the in the dark, I was very aware that the place would close for the weekend in less than an hour. I hammered, I kicked, I banged and thumped and sometimes I just lent against the wall and worried about how I could survive being stuck in there all weekend. To say my anxiety levels were high would be an understatement. It was about half an hour but felt like much, much longer. Finally the door opened and I was met with a small group of grinning and laughing faces – I found myself laughing with them, but deep down I was still very distressed and on the verge of tears. To this day I still have some issues with closed spaces and particularly, door handles and locks. In work we laugh about it from time to time and what happened this afternoon makes it funnier. The little staff kitchen has a handle that opens from both sides but when I was in there alone today it came off in my hand as I tried to leave. For a while disbelief and panic began to rise then I remembered that I'd been listening to music on my phone and had it with me. One phone call and someone was down in minutes to open the door. Again I found myself laughing at the absurdity of what had happened. We joked about how shit poor my luck was for it to have happened twice and I left as someone tried their best to re-secure the handle with the one and only screw that could be found. It WAS funny but I can't help feeling somewhat picked-on – after all, seriously, what are the odds that it would even happen? – let alone the same person! The emotions from years ago rushed back and I found it hard to play it down; I'd be embarrassed if they knew how much it actually freaked me out. For a few moments, until my mind settled, it felt just the same as before. Nobody's fault – just random bad luck. I may have been laughing about it with the guys but It helped that I'd made a bee-line for the diazepam the minute I'd got back to my desk. I'm gonna be checking door handles and locks now for the rest of my life – I knew I was right not to trust them. Seriously – never again."

Traffic lullaby

"Even as I cleared the last of the tea dishes from the table I was trying to decide how best, at only 8pm, to announce to my family that the day's holiday sightseeing had left me spent – that I needed to go to bed. I was drained: a day requiring little more than polite conversation and occasional smiles had been unbelievably challenging. I climbed into bed feeling pretty pleased with myself though – not only had I survived another difficult day but, as far as I knew, I'd done so without ruining anyone else's holiday. The little cottage backed on to the main road and for the longest time I just lay in the dark listening to the rhythm of the dwindling traffic as it passed purposefully by. The weather had been kind to us and the air was otherwise still and fresh as it crept into my room through a window left hopefully ajar. The night air is always welcome in my bedroom but doubly so when it is freshened by recent rain; it felt so good. This holiday came as I found myself in an episode of depression and at first I thought my mood would cast a shadow on my family's plans and I secretly wished I didn't have to go. As I lay there listening to the traffic I was all at once relieved and thankful and pleased that I did. When I had packed that holdall my depression hid between the t-shirts, there was no way I could have left it behind, but thankfully I had been able so far to keep it in check. My holiday remained my own. I didn't let it win."

Priorities

"I was off work yesterday because I felt so bad I literally couldn't get myself out of bed, but today I did get into work. (Cue dramatic music for the mini miracle.) It was a tough day and then, just when I thought it couldn't get any worse, I suddenly became VERY aware that I needed a shower. I mean REALLY needed a shower. I was annoyed at myself and felt even more useless than ever – how could I have let this happen again? Oh God, what must everyone around me have thought? The smell of stale sweat isn't exactly subtle after all. Was it noticeable? Was it my re-worn clothes? Was it me? How embarrassing. You see, most folk think depression is just about sitting in a dark corner wallowing in your own misery, but there can be practical aspects too. When I get depressed I lose all interest in 'personal grooming' I'll wear any random old clothes and for any number of days in a row. My hair often looks like you could fry chips in it, it's that greasy. I just don't care – after all, as far as I'm concerned, it's a miracle I'm out of my pyjamas at all. Now 'personal hygiene' – the thing is, it DOES suffer. But most of the time, when depressed, I really don't care – I do nothing at all, or if pushed, only the bare minimum. When I realised today that I was sat in work actually smelling quite strongly of stale sweat, I struggled to remember the last time I had showered or even brushed my teeth. When I'm depressed such things don't really exist. I just let everything go – after all – what's the point? Now here's another important thing – I'm relatively early into this depression and have pretty much been able to keep to my work routine. Because I was in my work when I noticed the problem I reacted quite sensibly but had I been deeper into my depression cycle, at home, lying around in my PJ's alone with just my dark thoughts for company, I probably wouldn't even have noticed – and if I did, I certainly wouldn't have given a damn! I know this because I've been there before. The further into depression I go, the less such issues even register. I am not alone in this. It is a common problem for depression sufferers and a source of great embarrassment once the mood begins to lift and we become aware of what we have been doing.

I did shower tonight when I got home but I can't say for sure I'll be able to keep up the effort. If I had 100 things on my priorities list right now, personal hygiene and grooming would fall somewhere about a 95."

It's a Wonderful Life

"When I was out on day release, I brought back this film so I could watch it in the lounge. Predictably, I got all weepy, but they weren't sad tears, they were happy tears. Watching this film made me realise I'd made the right choice – that life was worth living. Every time I am feeling low, or particularly if I'm nearing crisis, I watch this film – it's incredibly old and clichéd but it is so powerful they should hand out DVDs on prescription. *Shawshank Redemption* and the *Matrix* Trilogy are also in my top three, but this is the undisputed number one; this film has literally saved my life. Because I was watching it here in the lounge of a psych ward, it seemed all the more emotional. Ok, it's not the real world but it's a template for how the world could be."

You're not crazy

" 'Ok then, I'll see you in two weeks – and, you're **NOT** going crazy.' My CPN continued down the driveway towards her car and I was left on the doorstep, for the briefest of moments paralysed by the enormity of her parting words. I'm not crazy – such a relief. Today I had finally told her that I believed I had some form of OCD in addition to my other issues. Even after putting it in writing to my psychiatrist I was still uncomfortable talking about it and I stumbled my way through, all the while scared of how my words would be received. I was relieved to hear that what I was describing did sound like OCD and that she knew I wasn't imagining things. After all these years of hiding it and being embarrassed to admit to it, I recounted my 'OCD' experience in small steps, testing the waters before moving on; about 5 minutes into the conversation though, I began to feel more comfortable and less like a freak. I still consider it strange that I should be able to talk freely and in detail about suicidal ideation and yet feel the need to hide a compulsion to use door handles to influence the future, that I had bought into a stereotype and stigma – the very thing I have lately come to stand strongly against. In my mind all these years, my OCD labelled me a hopelessly frightened and stupid crazy person. This self-image sits in sharp relief to my more comfortable 'bipolar' identity; I've been pushing the OCD thing down, burying it and trying to pretend it didn't exist but this moment in time has presented itself as my best hope and these past few days I have begun, with tentative steps, to openly explore this strange part of me. My CPN said this is perfectly normal – that mental health treatment is like peeling an onion – as one issue, one layer, is dealt with and peeled away, another is exposed. She told me not to feel bad about hiding these things but to focus on the fact that I had now progressed to a point where I felt strong enough to finally deal with them. She reminded me that this is ultimately a good thing and that I wasn't going crazy after all. I so needed to hear that."

Nothing was said

"This Monday morning I sat at my desk chatting excitedly with the two girls standing to its right hand corner. There had been a party since we broke for the weekend and (T) was describing the detail of the fantastic three-tier birthday cake. Innocently, she flicked my filing tray around 45 degrees, and began to motion around it with her hands to indicate the dimension of the cake base. Exactly what she said, I couldn't tell you because I was totally consumed, staring at the tray – words of protest trapped behind gritted teeth. "Put the tray back... Put the tray back... Put the tray back," – but no, the tray was abandoned at its rakish angle as she went on to describe the seating arrangements. I needed to reach out and fix it, but I couldn't quite reach it without being obvious about it. (S) came to my rescue. Whilst chatting away, she gently touched her finger to the corner of the black tray and guided it back to parallel. I glanced up at her and was met with a little smile. Nothing was said."

Anxiety

"Sometimes I feel like the 'how' is irrelevant – I'm done for either way. I can stay in my bubble until it cracks and collapses in around me – or – I can allow myself to be pulled to the surface so quickly that I can't handle the change in pressure, and die from 'rescue'. What if I make it? What if I make my way to the surface and it's all too big, too loud, and too intense? Too scary? Maybe that kind of trapped would be worse! Maybe the world can't or won't accept me? Maybe I won't even be me anymore? What if I lose what made me me – I don't know how to be anyone else. Do I really need to change? Will the world ever change? Am I ready to risk another failure? My world is already changing. People are already treating me differently. A diagnosis is just another label for them to judge me by. Getting help may have made things worse."

{The main text fits over a sketch of a globe, not unlike a snow globe. At the base there is an unremarkable mountain surrounded by grass off to the horizon. It rises more than half way up the globe. The lines above it extend downward, almost to its peak and look like cracks in the outer globe or lightening within it depending on the point of view. To one side, beyond the globe, there are many angular doodle composed of intersecting straight lines. There is a recurring stair like theme.}

Again

"We talked for half an hour and now I struggle to recall what was said. It was much as many before it – a non-conversation. Like decorations that are pulled from the attic year after year, the words were notably tired and ill-suited to the job at hand. I had hoped for more, but my own words could not do justice to the indefatigable emptiness."

The small things

"I'm slipping into an episode of depression – at least I didn't get ambushed this time, I saw it coming and was able to do a few things to improve the situation a little – can't stop it happening but I can at least try to take the edge off. This evening I am taking time out to acknowledge some of the small positives in my day – to remind myself that it's not all about negativity and dark thoughts. 1: I actually did make it through the day – each one is a victory – one at a time. 2: I made it through a work day even though I felt really bad and could barely function. 3: I spent time with my family for a birthday celebration and I remembered how to smile. 4: I got a lovely long 'make it all better' hug from my husband – always great. 5: I got text messages from my best mate who is always encouraging me and supporting me. 6: I put on my first pair of 36 jeans in years – weight loss still on track; three sizes down now. 7: I had a bowl of cherries – love cherries. Always a treat. 8: My cleaner did a wonderful job at the house again tonight – I'd struggle without her. 9: I was able to listen to my favourite music most of the working day. 10: I have a comfy bed waiting for me in a safe house. I can rest well.

These seemingly small and insignificant things punctuated an otherwise dark and challenging day. I remember them now and acknowledge just how important the small things in life really are."

I don't need you to fix me

"I don't need you to 'fix' me. I just need to know you'll be there to support me while I try to work through all this crap. Yes, I'm depressed. Yes, our conversation probably did provide the spark. Things have moved on though – that spark is now a raging fire that is destined to cause severe damage before it burns itself out. You didn't start it. I didn't start it. Together though, if you can allow me to lean on you, we can perhaps contain it and limit the damage. Deep down I sort of knew an episode of depression was on the cards; one usually does come after the hypomania. Thing is, it really doesn't matter how prepared I think I am, I still get lost in the darkness, the thick smoke choking out the will to live. I don't need you to put the fire out – I need you to guide me through it – show me a reason to keep fighting – a reason not to curl up in the darkness and give up on life. I know I close off and it's difficult to talk sometimes but I still need your reassurance; I need your help; I need to know that you love me. I need to know you will listen without judging me, that you will believe the things I tell you. You told me once that trying to get close to me when I was depressed was like trying to hug an angry Rottweiler. For that I'm truly sorry, but I am the darkest version of myself when I'm depressed – because I'm hurting, I'm angry at the world, angry at myself, angry at everything – and all the while so incredibly tired of life itself and of trying to fit in and live the lie. I need you to know that now, more than ever; the small things are actually the most important. Don't try to fight the fire – because you can't; just show me a pathway out of it and be patient while I find the courage and strength to walk it. To find myself without you would be the final straw. Please don't leave me alone in there."

Stable

"I have to remind myself sometimes that it's ok to be stable, that I should rest and enjoy it; it's difficult though because the mood swings are ferocious beasts that contentment could ever hope to fight off. A strange paranoia creeps into my life and I am forever fearful of the shadows that dance among the routine and the unremarkable. They are coming for me... it's only a matter of time."

Macarena

"Dale a tu cuerpo alegria Macarena
Que tu cuerpo es pa' darle alegria cosa buena
Dale a tu cuerpo alegria, Macarena
Hey Macarena!
(Ay!)
Hey Macarena

Remember that tune? And let's face it, you SANG that in your head didn't you? – You didn't just read it. Remember how it ate into your brain and had you mumbling your way through a language you didn't even understand?

Hey Macarena!
Hey Macarena!

Tapping the steering wheel as you drove your car, fumbling in front of the bedroom mirror trying to get the dance moves down. Then finding yourself 'sing' it ment...

Hey, Dale a tu cuerpo alegria Macarena
Que tu cuerpo es pa' darle alegria cosa Buena

...ally in the gaps between other thoughts. It really did

Hey, Dale a tu cuerpo alegria Macarena
Que tu cuerpo es pa' darle alegria cosa Buena

begin to take over – It became the soundtrack to you day just because you heard it on the radio whilst eating cornflakes. It was insidious. It was intr...

Hey, Dale a tu cuerpo alegria Macarena
Que tu cuero es pa' darle alegria cosa Buena

...usive and unwelcome by midday and totally freaked you out when you lay your head down at night to sleep only to find it playing and playing and playing in your mind – louder and louder – faster and faster –

and you STILL didn't even understand it.

Hey, Macarena!! Hey, Dale a tu cuerpo alegria Macarena, Que tu,
Hey Macarena!!

It got to the point it wasn't even making sense.

Do you remember?

If you do, then perhaps you have small insight into my mind because lately 'dark thoughts' have been my Macarena. That's about as close as I can get to explaining the way they eat into my brain.

HEY MACARENA!!"

Workday thoughts

"Elbows on the table, eyes softly closed as outstretched fingers massage the temples in deliberate, soothing circles before brushing with pressure into the hair. I take off my glasses and hold them in my right hand as the left rubs tired eyes. I'm not tired – well, not in a physical sense – sleep is not what I'm craving. I just need to be alone with this aching mental exhaustion – somewhere that quietly exists on the edge of daily life – somewhere where I can drop the charade and perhaps begin to deal with the emotional cloud that has hung over me all day. I want to take time off work and retire to my bed where I feel safe. I want to hug the pillow tight and curl up in foetal comfort, but my stronger self keeps talking me into going to work. Yet again I have found myself at my desk, surrounded by stuff I can't begin to process. Other people's urgencies are ill-attended when my thoughts have to struggle through treacle and I almost gag on the emotions trying to escape my heavy, heavy body. I need to vent – I can't. When eight hours are passed and the twelve-hour shift is done, I pause expectantly but no words acknowledge my mammoth effort nor, hands outstretch to pat me on the back or offer up a hug. I used to think that no one cared but actually, I know there are many who do; my sense of invisibility is born of their misunderstandings and my own inaction. When I'm being stalked by depression, the harder I fight to fend it off, the more 'well' I seem. The more 'well' I seem, the less likely I am to receive support because no one can see through the vacant smile and see the girl struggling with demons. I'm reluctant to draw attention. It's my fault."

Rough, raw and swollen

"I don't have dry mouth today – I have 'dry tongue' It's the weirdest thing. Any time before that my lovely meds cocktail has delivered dry mouth, it's had the decency to do the gums, the palette – but not the tongue! God, it's annoying beyond belief – rough and raw and swollen and screaming at me every time it makes contact to eat or talk. Water makes f**k all difference because I've always drunk litres a day, the pastilles and gels work a little on the normal stuff, but nothing works on the tongue. I even tried toothpaste. So, telling myself that it's not that bad, that it will pass. I'm putting up with it because the antipsychotic I'm taking now is so much better than the old one. I'm a little more 'mellow' but not 'dazed' and the rotten side effects I'd had with the old stuff are gone. My bl**dy period came back though, which was admittedly a bit of a bummer after five years of freedom. Still, you can't have everything. Dry mouth, dry tongue, whatever – I've only just got my meds sorted out and I don't want to go upsetting the apple cart by complaining again to my CPN."

My best mate

"I have this mate; my best mate. He's a he, which I know is somewhat unusual but even though we'll never go shopping together for shoes, he remains my closest friend. Has been for years. This isn't based on being 'joined at the hip' because we actually don't see each other that often. He holds a special place in my heart because of how he makes me feel when we are together – we communicate mainly by laughter and hugs, but he is also fluent in shared silence. We've helped each other through some intensely difficult times – shared some deeply personal stuff. He totally accepts me for who I am and isn't ever afraid to give me a reality check when I need one. Once, after I'd been in an armed robbery and was sat at home scared, remembering what it felt like to have a gun held to my head, so scared they were coming back for me, he came round and sat watching hours of chick flicks that he hated, just to make me feel safe until my husband came home. I rang him once when I was feeling suicidal and he was at my door in minutes. We talk about things like how 42 is the answer to life, the universe and everything and what would happen if you put soap in a microwave. He makes me laugh when he quotes my favourite bits verbatim from *Blackadder* or *Red Dwarf*. A lot of people would take him for a tough guy but, although I know he'd never hesitate to step in to defend me from harm, I also know he has a pure and gentle heart. I love my husband – I love my mate – and most of all, I love that we're all friends; we grew through our formative years together. I trust him without question and I know he actually means it when he says he will always be there for me. He makes me smile and makes me feel good about myself. He scares away the demons and reminds me there is good in this world. His name is Dean. Without him I may not have survived this long."

The girl in the mirror

"The weight of judgement hung heavy around me like a thick woollen coat at the height of summer. Stifling. I'd carried it for so long I'd begun to think I'd never be able to shake it off. I not only listened to other people's opinion of me and how I lived with my bipolar illness, I started to live it as truth. Everyone I spoke to had a different label to pin to my chest and I began to believe them – I felt I had come as far as was possible and I was destined to live out my days as the moody, attention-seeking weirdo. One day I dug up some self-confidence and decided I was done being a piñata for other people's judgements and I was going to figure out just who I really was and what my diagnosis had to do with it all anyway. I hadn't a clue where to start but knew things had to change and I was going to have to be the one to make those changes. I looked in the mirror and didn't recognise the girl looking back at me; I was afraid and confused and anxious most of the time but she seemed so much calmer – normal almost. And so began the chase…I wanted to find out what she had that I didn't. The biggest truth that I tripped over on my journey was that my illness does NOT define me. I accept it now as a big part of me, and a part I would not even erase if given the choice. Once that truth filtered through me I found I was already more comfortable in my own skin. I still encountered judgements around me, but instead of letting them cling to me and squeeze my spirit, I brushed them off as best I could. Stigma is everywhere and I have accepted that many of the people I encounter will resort to judgement out of ignorance and fear: occasionally I have felt the sting of pure malice but thankfully not that often. Nowadays, I hold no grudge. I have made the difficult decision to be as open and honest as possible about my bipolar disorder and self harm. There has been a difficult transition in work since my diagnosis, but I've managed to hold down my full time job and the routine, social interaction and sense of contribution underpin my continued stable state. When I get home I am totally exhausted physically and especially mentally, but I don't beat myself up any more about my inability to function as a perfect housewife. I have accepted my limitations and the trade off: I get help now at home and that allows me to direct all my energy and purpose into a positive working day. I learn as much as possible about my illness, treatments etc. The cocktail of coping strategies I now employ keeps me surfing the wave rather than becoming overwhelmed and drowning. Nothing is 100% effective and what works one week will not necessarily work the next but I am learning to use each one where and when I feel it would be most effective and I'm genuinely proud of how well I've been doing lately. Yes, I still get the mood swings and the pervading thoughts of self harm and suicide but not as I used to. We all travel our own journey and all have our experiences in trying to find balance. This year I have found a group of coping strategies that work for me. Journaling and mood tracking combine for me into a hybrid spreadsheet tool – I record everything of significance and being able to look back through the data gives unique insight. I have learnt by trial and error which meds work best for me and I try really hard to ensure I do actually take them as I should. I take every opportunity afforded me to speak with my key workers; I've learnt a lot from them and value their ability to listen without judgement. Good sleep/medication patterns are absolutely essential. Regular recreational activity is difficult for me, especially given the social anxiety but I do what I can and it really does help me stay stable. I know there would be a lot of people wary of using meditation or breathing techniques but I find them both invaluable. I get tremendous peer support from Twitter and have been privileged to be able to help some others in their moment of crisis. Of course there is now the wonderful emotional outlet called blogging. This year, I was referred for Cognitive behavioural therapy. It taught be to recognise a forming negative thought and to challenge it. The principal is very simple but the payoff is fantastic. I use it every day. My depressions would often cripple me for many weeks, but my last one only lasted four; I was even functioning well enough to keep working. Because I am open with family, friends and work colleagues, I am so lucky to be able to talk freely when I hit a difficult patch and I am forever grateful that the weight of secrecy has been lifted from my shoulders. I talk a lot, in the world around me and that of social media. It is my release valve. I'm lucky to have it. Finally, there is the issue of self harm. At the time of writing this, I have not turned to self harm in over three months. Guided by the idea of the butterfly project, I place a temporary tattoo of a butterfly close to the area I'd normally harm; simply then, the challenge is to refrain from harming while the butterfly remains intact. When I feel the need I can call on the butterflies. It's not perfect – but it's good. As coping strategies go, I've collected quite a mixed bag and these are just some of the things tested in my experience and proving their worth time and time again. Lately, when I look in the mirror, I don't see a stranger: I see myself. The chasing is over but the journey continues."

The bookcase was shouting at me

"It was just wrong. Wrong. Wrong in the way a flat note in the middle of your favourite song is wrong. I could see that bookcase out of the corner of my eye and my skin crawled as the discomfort seeped out of every pore. I could take it no longer – the mess just had to go! I had to make it right; I had to be ruthless. My own bookcase sits to my left – It is the picture of perfect order, everything millimetre square and labelled to ensure nothing could end up in the wrong place. The notice board behind me has more personal items than work ones but those photos and quotes help keep my mind in the right place – these too, are carefully pinned to follow the mental grid I impose on the cork base. My desk is just as it should be. Drawer units and filing trays are blu-tacked down to stop them shifting from the parallel: the sheets inside are always in the top left corner. Staplers, tape, pen trays etc are all sitting in the exact place they should be sitting – and I mean exactly – and that holepunch is on its side and facing the door. My notebook has no spaces – empty space is just wrong – I write in a continuous string. When I'm working on stuff, I have out only the bare minimum of paperwork and I keep it in a neatly tapped in pile. I work one line, one page, one item at a time – systematically – to my own system, mentally ticking off the stages as I go. I like my desk. It is exactly as it needs to be and when I know the cleaner has been in on Wednesday mornings, I enter with trepidation because millimetres matter. I can't start my working day until everything on my desk is exactly where it should be so you can imagine how the peripheral sight of that dumping ground of a bookcase nearby was upsetting me. I stripped it and ruthlessly binned all but the essentials: I dusted it down and squared off all the files. Now, it's pretty much perfect because there are even two empty shelves – Yay! It took only 20 minutes and now I can settle into my work routine again without it shouting at me. I am aware that others around me find my behaviour a little odd; I am aware that this behaviour an example of mild OCD tendencies. Strange thing is – I am not like this at home. I don't adjust ornament into correct position 15mm away. I don't square off all the books on my own bookcase. Ok, some of the knives have a specific place on the magnetic board and some toiletries have their own specific spot on the bathroom unit and I do have this thing about door handles wherever I go but my home life isn't otherwise informed by such rules. The world of work is difficult for me to deal with – the social issues – stress – the politics – the concentration issues – memory issues- mood issues – distraction – uncertainty – tiredness – all that crap. I have simply found a way to cope. My little constructed world protects me and helps me perform. I don't care that it's the OCD. What harm is it doing anyone? The only casualty lately has been that bookcase and I'm pretty sure everyone else in the office was pretty pleased to finally see it done."

Of course words can harm

"Sticks and stones may break my bones, but words can never harm me -
Who the f**k are they trying to kid? Of course words can harm! Hell, words can kill! The truth informs even those words that seek to hide behind humour or sarcasm – the delicate heart can divine

underlying truth because in repetition it becomes more recognisable – the delicate heart weeps silent tears and bids the mind to not engage. To muddy the waters further and stir up the pain would achieve little.

And the dream, of course, is to somehow return to the clear waters; to a time when words warmed the heart and touched the soul."

Challenging a self harm trigger

"Dark thoughts often come uninvited, but occasionally they arrive when the door is left ajar by an innocent word, smell, object – trigger. Today, in fact for many days now, I've been doing great. I feel about as stable as I ever get to feel and life seems less of a personal challenge. Things are good. This afternoon though, one of those split-second, ambush-you-from-out-of-nowhere triggers came at me – screamed so loud at me that I just couldn't ignore it. It got inside my head and resurrected a bundle of feelings so jumbled that I almost caught myself panic. A few shards of broken glass resting on a carpeted cutting bench. That's all. They had no doubt been there since the picture framing department closed over a year ago and as the room was now little more than a corridor to other places, what need had there ever been to sweep them up? They were harmless. I was easily 12 feet away but I could clearly see the sharp edges of the clustered pieces contrasted against that dirty brown – in fact, for a moment, it was all I could see. How could I not have noticed them before? Memories of previous cuts came rushing at me with an intensity I had not expected and the trigger lived up to its name. All of a sudden, my head was full of images best not described here in detail; my mind was besieged by thoughts trying to justify them. In that split second I found myself wanting to cut again – I so wanted to. But, to my credit, I turned 90 degrees and headed for the double doors and down into the warehouse. I walked its length slowly and then took a detour outside through the loading bays, all the while trying to regain my composure. By the time I walked back into the offices I was ok and my afternoon continued as if nothing had ever happened. It does happen though. More often than you would think. I can't control the triggers but I'm trying to control how I deal with them. Just another day as me."

Miss you Furball

"Krissy, wherever you are, I hope you are happy. I want to believe that you are well and have found another family to love. I need to believe that. I miss you so much. You are my friend, my counsellor, perhaps in a way my child. There's a part of me that will always ache for you. Your love was unconditional and you always sensed my pain and would come with your own special comfort. I want to feel your face brush my face and rub away the tears. I feel so lost without you. I'm angry they lost you. I won't believe you are dead. I won't accept that you're injured or hurting. You're alive and well and right now looking up from the lap of someone else who really needs you. Be happy. Make them happy – and please – forgive me for not saying goodbye. Please don't ever believe that I abandoned you. B'Elanna misses you still, but I know we'll work it out and be happy again. Thanks Krissy, for everything. Goodbye.
(Krissy by the way, is a cat. My cat. I left her in kennels while on holiday and they lost her – let her go! B'Elanna is her daughter.)"

Loneliness and tears

"I've just spent the better part of a lovely sunny Saturday scanning photos from old, old albums into folders on my laptop where all the other stuff lives. It took exactly one *War of the World*, two *Joseph*s and *Little Shop of Horrors* up to the bit where the dentist dies from an OD of laughing gas – in other words, hours! My head hurts and I'm stiff and a little sore, but I've made headway now into a project that's been on the 'to do' list for at least two years. Better late than never, eh? I'm feeling really sad though. Crying, actually. That social circle I'm always talking about, missing so badly – the one that dwindled away almost overnight and left me all alone feeling unwanted and unworthy – well it ambushed me more than once from the pages of those old dusty albums. Taunting me. Photo after photo of laughing faces; most particularly, photos with me in amongst it all. I never appreciated back then what a special thing it is to be surrounded by friends, to have parties, camping trips and days out at the beach. I know I have social anxiety. I know I have a mood disorder. I also know, however, that I'd give almost anything to be back in the middle of one of those parties, to have my circle of friends about me and feel a part of something again. That's why New Year and Christmas are always so dreadfully depressing and dangerous for me. The way other people's happiness hangs in the air like a thick fog is overpowering – It clouds my vision and fills my lungs until I suffocate. It can see right through my practiced smiles and targets me specifically. Now, just like then, I find myself helpless and tears are my only recourse. Loneliness, sadness, anger, self pity, rejection, shame, regret and painful loss all roll up into a second skin that I must carry with me every day. It hasn't left me in years but days like today make it so much worse. It must have been my fault and I wish so much I knew what I did wrong so I could go back and fix it. I miss them all. I miss the me I was when I was around them, part of them."

Radio

"I wanted to kill it. If I'd had a sturdy knife I'd have driven it into it and made it shut up... But instead, the factory floor radio went on and on and on... discussing suicide and the why's and wherefores and it made me want to scream. Thinking about it is bad enough, but everywhere I go it's on the TV, on the radio? It's stalking me! I put my earphones in and tried to listen to Classic FM, but it was all still there in the background, clear as day. I wanted to get away, get out of there – but where? I tried to think of somewhere I could be alone and have a good cry. I ended up in the toilets – not ideal I know, but that lock gave me the space I needed – I didn't have to come out until I was ready. Talk about it people say, be honest they say, be open they say, it will help they say – but how the hell do I explain this? I'm such a mess."

Chameleon

"Ear-plugs, sunglasses + squishy huggy pillow... Gently rocking, barely moving.... I tried to merge into the corner. I wanted to disappear. I love my family. I love my little nephews, but the noise makes me want to scream and run from the room. I can't decide whether I want to cry or scream; I'd have given just about anything for 10 minutes of silence! I move inward. I rock and find my own rhythm. I hear it all, but it is like I have shifted dimensions – there, but not quite there. I pull myself into a quieter place. I had to before I exploded. Beginning to feel like hedgehogging again – live in bed for a few days. Not coping that well at the minute."

Betrayal

"Too hurt to even go into details. The promised support was just a lie. Betrayal is a difficult thing to come to terms with. I keep thinking about that song "The Ballad of Glencoe". Yep, feels like that."

Start of the day

"9.00am – It took 3 alarms + a LOT of willpower to get me out of
bed this morning. I did wash my hair, but that was about all. I
grabbed some clothes from the 'everything matches' pile over the
banister and half awake went downstairs to feed the cat. 20mins
later my eyes still wanted to shut and I felt uncomfortably warm. I
went up stairs to get something but half way up forgot what it was; I
felt groggy. Half an hour later I opened the mail and read a letter
from my American pen pal. It began "Just touching base to see how
you are." Then he immediately it moved into "I went here, I did this,
blah blah blah" I skipped the odd line but read enough to know he
never actually DID ask how I was or make any reference to the
crisis I'd just lived through. It was dismissed amid the niceties of a
non-letter. What was the point? Why did he write if he didn't want to
actually have a conversation? I feel hurt. He probably thought it
best not to mention it so as not to make me feel bad but to totally
ignore me was so much worse. I just want to curl up and cry."

Sexual identity

"Love – Comfort – Togetherness – Fun – Intimacy – Confusion –
Change – Fantasies – Needs – Release -Escape – Sharing –
Playfulness – Friendship etc, etc. He's the better part of me. I love
him with everything it is in me to give. I'm lucky. I have a Hubby
who is loving and gentle and considerate and understanding.
Cuddles and hugs are always there when I need them and we've
enjoyed a very healthy sex life. However in the past, because of the
damn bipolar, I've gone through oscillating periods of disinterest
and insatiability with alarming frequency – it's been a real
rollercoaster ride. Lately I'm beginning to worry that the bipolar
meds are going to make things worse – my libido is fading. There's
enough uncertainty and challenge in our lives – I really don't want
to introduce more. Maybe things will settle? They should. I'm
probably worrying needlessly."

{Doodles of hearts and question marks}

The perpetuating kiss

"7am – a lazy half stretch is quickly followed by a yawn muffled with
duvet. So the world went and woke me up again did it? So much for
hibernation! I suppose I should open my eyes, well half open. Ok
then, reality check.... My own room, this is good. That must have

been a dream after all. I slap my hand around the bedside cabinet in search of the phone; the alarm seems unnecessarily loud but at least I'm awake...hold on a minute, is this good? What day is it anyway? Sure? ...? Right, better think about getting up then.....how am I feeling anyway? Is this a day for facing the world? 'Stop arguing you lot, I'll make up my own mind' Are you sure it's a work day? Oh f**k it then, let's give it a go. Hey look at me – I'm up – the words trail off – the mattress bounces slightly as I land back down unannounced. My eyes roll shut again as I curl foetally and wish the world away. My room means my bed and my bed is still warm and inviting. The fog of disturbed sleep begins to clear and my depression emerges; it tucks me in, places a kiss on my forehead with whispers that it's ok, that it will protect me from the reality of living. As I drift into waking dreams, it makes real its promises: today is not a day to face the world. Today is silently cursed in fact, just for having me in it."

Debate

"Found myself thinking things through in the darkness. Which would be best? Which would be quickest? Which would be least painful? Which easier on those left behind? Two hours ago I was watching Tom & Jerry – well trying to; I wasn't thinking like this. OD? Cut? Drown? Jump? On and on... as matter of fact as choosing a filling for a sandwich. Why do I do this to myself? I'm so screwed up. I can't even cry any more. What's wrong with me? This sux."

My little red squishy

"It's a pillow/mini beanbag kinda thing; bought @ an air show as a practical cushion, but now it's been transformed – it's a portable hug! For some reason – and no, I don't really know why, it's now my comforter – like a 2yr old with a 'blanky'. I rarely go anywhere without it these days; I even sleep with it. I cuddle it + play with it, kneading and squishing when I'm feeling really low or panicky. I know I embarrass people when I carry it with me around town or in shops, but right now; I need it – especially in crowds and other scary stressful places. I get unbelievably jittery. I notice myself beginning to sway, my hands get all clenchy + tappy; sometimes my foot starts sorta twitching and I almost hold my breath in anticipation of a panic attack that may never come."

3am again

"I'm getting quite used to the cold, dark silence of 3am; we're pals
now. Even the clocks tick seems to be saying, "Go to sleep, go to
sleep, go to sleep," but I can't. I can snuggle. I can close my eyes –
but sleep – no. Oh, how I wish for one of those 'can hardly stay
awake' days. I'd take them – bad dreams an' all right now. I'm wide
awake but just can't make any real use of the time – it is SO
frustrating! If it wouldn't freak everyone out to find me gone, I'd just
up and go – walk the roads for some fresh air and see the sky. But
I'm staying with Mum and Dad and the house is already full of
worries – they'd panic. TV is no company at a time like this + I can't
concentrate enough to read. Guess it's just me + my anxiety until 4
or 5 when maybe I might be able to do doze off. It's at this shitty
hour of the morning I usually feel most alone, and at my most
vulnerable – it's only me and the empty night."

Nothing

"Not one card or visit – not even a bunch of flowers from a garage!
The only contact by phone was initiated by me – they certainly
weren't about to call. Crazy isn't contagious! I can understand why
they're behaving like this but that doesn't stop it stinging like hell.
Why are they avoiding me? Am I a lost cause? I guess I'm
expecting too much, even from friends."

Thought charts

{Four A4 pages full of thought charts all done in the space of
10mins – the pencil could hardly keep up and the writing is close to
unreadable. There are circled words splitting and linking into other
circled words and phrases; lines franticly drawn all over the place to
connect groups of circles. Looking as messy and confused as the
mind the churned them out – lots of question marks and no
answers visible.}

Said in innocence

"I could just kill myself... The words latched on the trailing sentence
and hung in the air just long enough to raise an expected laugh.
Why were they laughing? How is that funny? He said it in
innocence; he had no idea the demons he was summoning – I

choked down words of protest and instead retired to another room, there to begin dealing with the summoned darkness."

Hugs

"Been staying with Mum and Dad most nights because Hubby had to work. The days can be hard as the kids are about – it's so noisy sometimes, but at least its company, it's routine. Last night I plunged into one of those 'dark hopeless, cry for everything yet nothing' times. I rocked and I cried and tried to fight my way through it. I got scared. I didn't want to be alone so I went to Mum's room, woke her up and told her I needed a hug. Me, a 39-year-old, I went to Mummy for a hug. It's a really good job I wasn't alone at home. Now, this morning the thoughts of suicide are melting into the ether and although I totally look like crap, I feel so much better. I actually got properly dressed and I'm ready to try and face the world. (Still carrying that hidden blade though – but one day at a time, one thing at a time)."

Pink

"I used to joke that sometime before I reached 40, I was going to dye my hair shocking pink – just for the fun of it. Never really knew why, but the idea appealed to me. Right now, I SO want to do it. Of course everyone would think I was crazy – but then I am – so is that good or bad? No one reacted badly when I went from waist-long hair to shaved and permed bob in one appointment. Why should they care if I go pink? Why should I care if they care or not? Tempting."

Emerging pearl

"The lustre and sheer beauty of a pearl is born of turmoil and decay – the unending cycle of the waters providing all that is required. As the waters wash in and around the oyster nestling in its shell, the grit swirls about and begins to accumulate until it builds in a crescendo of splendour. But what is it really? Waste – byproduct – natural discharge; we adorn ourselves with waste. What I'm trying to say is – beauty is relative. Appreciation is relative. All things are relative. In moments of meditation I often consider whether I am in fact the oyster or the pearl. Most often I am the pearl, cast of grit waiting to grow into something more worthwhile. The waters that sustain me tease with hints of a larger world but I for now remain trapped in the shell. At times the shell is my protection but even as it rises in the moonlight it is at once my prison; I am conflicted. Is that larger world really a better place?"

Mess

"My house is a mess! Untouched, undisturbed. Basically living away from home because I can't risk being alone. In a flurry of activity and energy I can clean, tidy and clear + organise here, but not my own house! At home I can't settle; it's better that I'm here. It's 3.27am and it feels like lunch time – nothing new there

What's real?

"(Complete panic. My heart is trying to push out of my chest and I can hardly breathe, let alone talk. I'm desperately frustrated and at the end of my rope. I'm trying to convince a reluctant 999 operator to get me to a hospital…then just like that I'm there but they won't take me in. I can't remember what crisis prompted the call, I KNOW I have to get in, that it's my only hope. No one listens. They patronise me then ignore me and the panic shifts up a step. I'm screaming, consumed by utter panic; I NEED to get in) … And then I guess I woke up. Everything was a bit foggy for a moment and my heart was still doing somersaults. I was breathing quick and shallow and I was still drenched in panic. My foot was doing that twitching thing too. I was overwhelmed so reached for the pad and pen beside my bed and started to scribble this... to try and reinforce reality and ease the residual fear and panic. I can hear the cat purring but even that seems faster than usual. I can't write quickly enough. I feel sick in the stomach. God, why won't that foot stop tapping? I can't keep up. Need to stop."

Hey, look at me...

"I'm going to a rock tribute show tomorrow night and to crowded IKEA on Sunday. I'm going to the cinema on Monday for a charity screening of my favourite film and I'm quite impressed that I find myself up to it all, one day after the other. I was at a function Friday past and survived well despite some rising anxiety. I'm determined to keep trying as I want to be able to get out there and enjoy Christmas this year; it's been three years from I've even put a tree up."

Bubbles

"Visiting hours are over. I spent them alone, quietly writing and gathering my thoughts. I just finished a somewhat philosophical journal on the nature of identity and was about to put it all away when someone thoughtfully placed a cup of tea on my table. It was full of bubbles, which my superstitious Gran used to say foretold coming wealth. I thought of her for quite some time and replayed some old memories. I was still quite young when she died but I still think of her. Why now? I don't know. Perhaps I just summoned her from my subconscious to raise a smile. My memory may increasingly let me down with faces, names, processes and stuff but never has it failed me when it comes to something like this.

Pill panic

"The family talked me into going away for a weekend hotel break. Agreed. Realised was almost out of diazepam + needed my sick line renewed so after a couple of days trying to remember, I finally rang the doctor to order them and some other stuff. Dad picked it up the morning we were to leave + came back with everything they'd ordered, everything that is but the diazepam! They'd left it off the prescription. Only had ONE left. Couldn't think of going without it so had to ring the doc and the chemist to try and sort it out. I was edgy and worried. I could feel myself getting all wound up and panicky. Caught myself swaying. May not use them much but just HAD to have them. Had to know they'd be there. By the time I got the bottle, I had to take one but I haven't needed one since. The diazepam are my security blanket – if I carry them I feel better. I don't use them unless I really have to – promised the doctor I'd be careful. Does it make me weak that I need them so? It hardly matters – it is what it is."

Four in the morning

"It's four in the morning, and once more the dawning, has wok… oh, drifting into an old country and western song there – where did that come from? It's four in the morning. My mind has been racing all day. 1st good night's sleep in months last night – a one-hour nap this afternoon + all day this… It won't stop. Thoughts all over the place and I can't focus. Feel edgy. Tried the internet to distract but no good. Tried TV but couldn't follow it at all – pausing, channel hopping – no good. Need some company – Sometimes the hyper days are worse than the sad ones."

Real but not real

"When I woke this morning I remembered almost every detail of the weird…well I suppose…dream…. But I'm not really sure. What was troubling was something that I 'saw' not dreamt – well at least I'm convinced I saw her but it may have been a trick of twilight sleep? I was awake – was just lying there – warm – comfy. As real as this pencil and pad right now – I lay in bed in the dimness and felt Krissy playfully clawing at my exposed foot at the end of the bed. As I always did, I pulled in and she rubbed and walked her way up to lie at my chest – curled in tight after much padding and preparing. She settled and I lay stroking her; she looked at me with her best 'ain't I cute' face and nudged up to lie nose to nose. I could see her – feel her – feel the vibration of her purr. It was real – at least as real as I can determine now – it didn't feel like a dream – it was real. Problem is – I stayed in a hotel last night and Krissy has been missing since the Kennels lost her months ago. Now, either I'm dreaming in a weird way or I'm seeing things that couldn't possibly be there. I'm worried – even though it was a comforting something – something isn't right. How do I know what's real? I'm still convinced I saw her but how could I have?"

Curl up

"For some reason, can't stand noise today? Motorbikes whizzing round the track while Hubby watches his races and it's driving me mad. An irritating, whining, non-stop sort of noise. Later the volume goes down again because *Sponge Bob* was on (normally like it) but his voice is so high-pitched and chirpy – Urghhhh – annoying much? TV normally sits around 18/20 but no matter what's been on so far today I've tried to get it muted or @ 3 or 4. I don't want to talk much – not in the mood for 20 questions. I just want to curl up and do the hedgehog thing. Sometimes when I want to curl up, I just need some space, some quiet time; sometimes I just want to curl up and sleep and never wake up?? Need to go @ my own pace… Need to feel safe… Need to be able to hide… Need to be able to rest… Need to stay close to the ground… I'm only gonna open up when I feel safe – I CAN only risk opening up when I feel safe. I've had too many bad experiences. I'm on the lookout for a big pile of autumn leaves to snuggle up in."

{Four little drawings of hedgehogs of various sizes, two of which are bedded in a pile of leaves.}

Even though...

"Even though I have recently decided to be open about my mental illness, there are still some conversations I don't really want to have; it's not because I have difficulty talking – it's because they have difficulty understanding, and I'm still learning the best ways to explain things. The problem is mine not theirs. Hopefully it will get easier

The pad

"I keep a notepad and pencil beside my bed and one in my handbag. It means I can jot down stuff that comes into my mind and I don't have to worry about remembering it; it's very freeing. It's also good if a poem decides to try and write itself."

Butterflies

"I was so upset I climbed into bed, curled up and cried myself to sleep. I've just woken up – about 3 hours later; eyes are all stingy + sore head is heavy + tummy is being gnawed at from the inside. I've got really bad wind – can't stop burping and belching and it's annoying. It happens when I'm really upset. Guess my 'butterflies' are more active than most. Maybe it's a throw back to my yoga training? Maybe I'm just more sensitive to the body/mind connection? Anyway, I have about another hour of this to look forward to until it finally settles."

{Detailed drawings of two delicate butterflies.}

Barometer

"I've realised that appointment dates are a good barometer of how well the professionals think you are doing. They all do it and I can't believe I hadn't noticed before. The longer the gap between appointments, the better they think you're coping. Obvious. Really, how stupid was I not to have noticed that?"

Pendulum

"The pendulum drops from hypomania and swings right through 'stable' on the way to depression. Back and forth with purposeful momentum – from one extreme to the other – passing through 'stable' as if it were not even there. It occurs to me that I do the same thing with this journal – I write to exorcise demons or to find stillness, but rarely to pause and write about the gift of stability. Normal days, if I dare call them that, are by definition unremarkable but I should make more of an effort to acknowledge them. When I read this journal back I want it to remind me that my bipolar self also occupied middle ground – that stability was a reality."

Inverse side effects

"My medication side effects are all confused – they don't happen when I take the stuff, they happen when I don't! It's the weirdest thing, but I've finally made the connection – there's one tablet, an anti-psychotic – all I have to do is skip one evening dose, just one, and it claims cruel revenge. About 12 hours later I begin to develop horrendous dry-mouth; the upper palette gets dry and rough, the rest of the mouth gets uncomfortable and I get little sores on the already painful tongue where it catches in the teeth. When I first started taking it, the dry mouth thing was an active side effect. It drove me mad for a long time before it became manageable, acceptable, but this 'revenge tactic' is quite annoying. I will however live with it because that little tablet is doing a great job in every other way. It's all about compromise."

Good day

"Today was a good day. This week has been a good week. This month has been a good month. I don't usually write about the good days because they are comfortable and happy and less intense. I should though, in the interest of balance, but they'll probably escape record because I'm too busy enjoying them to write about them."

Pencils and not pens

"Pens are too slow – can't keep up with my head. Pencils are better, quicker. Computer is quicker still but not always around + somehow it's not the same. Pencils are quicker, but even pencils can't keep up. My fingers sometimes hurt from holding too tight and I know I shouldn't grip like that but I get tense as I try to get it all down on paper. I can't write neatly. I haven't time to spell right and I just don't care. I feel like it's my pressure valve – no – I'm sure of it. I've always written and it has always helped, even if it doesn't always make sense. I've long since thrown away many old journal sheets. I wish I hadn't. Wish they were there to look back on."

{A large drawing of a sharpened pencil and repeatedly, the word 'Help'.}

Voices

"I hear voices in my head, well – sort of – there are lots of them but they are all me – it's weird. They gave up talking long ago and now they just whisper or shout. They all say different things – present different perspectives – have different questions – have different answers. They are all their own little personalities yet they are all me! I'm so messed up – what's going on? I've lost the little angel and devil on the shoulder that everyone has – the rational, balanced, binary guidance, and now I have so many voices I feel like my head is going to implode. The whisper plays cat and mouse, toying with me, invading my dreams and eating away at me slowly. I long for silence but even there the whisper can find me. They are all me. They are all my voice – every one of them – so why can't I make them leave me alone? Are they all real or just the one who is talking now? I can't trust my thinking or my judgement because I know they are compromised. Ironic really – that I should complain so bitterly about how others have betrayed me and yet I betray myself."

Random thoughts on yoga

"I miss yoga. Yoga was 'Me time' … Body, mind and spirit are one… Communion… Love…..Truth…. Gratitude…. Union… Peace… Balance… Belonging… Trust… Beauty… Stillness… Motion & Emotion & Inspiration as one…True peace need not be hunted down; it rests in the pause between breaths. It is always there, always available to us…"

Bouncing

"I woke this morning with what felt like the mother of all headaches... I couldn't lift my head... Physically and mentally it felt like there was destruction derby going on in there. There were so many thoughts + feelings colliding that I couldn't even really make sense of it. It felt like something was actually bouncing off the inside of my head. I felt uneasy, jittery, and nervous – could only lie there and wait until the bouncing subsided. Then I went downstairs + took my tablets. That's how my day started. I've been up about 2½ hours now, but it's definitely a hedgehog day."

{Drawing of a box with lots of little balls bouncing about and movement lines too.}

2.33am

"I miss my Hubby. He's been away all week driving + I've barely seen him. Txt + calls just aren't the same. I need a hug. I need to talk. I'll see him tomorrow – well today technically... but right now I need him. I'm thinking about Monday when I'm due to go to the psych ward for a while. I'm nervous – maybe even a little scared. He's my anchor – the reason I never quite acted on any of those plans. He's the one I need right now and I can't even ring him 'cause he'll be asleep. Thinking about our midnight picnics by the river – or even that time on the beach. The whole place to ourselves, cuddling in the night air + watching the sea creep along. I wish we were there right now. I need to cuddle. I even miss that silly grin he pulls just to bug me. I wonder is he dreaming of me?"

Asteroid

"I haven't been able to get to sleep and now it's morning – those folk on TV last night were explicit about the hows and whys an asteroid is destined to collide with earth and the horrendous aftermath that would ensue. Some even dared to forecast a date. The quiet voice that tried to sooth my nerves was angrily shouted down by those that accepted the inevitable truth. I have been playing the what-ifs over and over in my head all night, literally all night, and those images were not easy to look at. Anxiety is what I do best. I try to rein it in but it takes on a frightening life of its own and I am soon consumed by it. Last night was no exception and even now, as I prepare to face the new day, that anxiety stirs up a current of discomfort. Free from last night's onslaught, the lone voice of reason dares to speak again; it tells me not to be taken in, not to worry about things that are beyond my control. It tells me to calm down – if only it was that easy. I don't want to talk about this – people would think me foolish and laugh. I can't control it. My anxiety doesn't have an off switch, even if the root of it is something quite outrageous, unreasonable or unlikely."

Identity

"I am what I am, but that is always in flux. Here or there, or sharing the same space in two different dimensions... I sometimes wonder which is worse – co-existence or merging? Will I disappear? Who will the new me be? Will I like her? Maybe we should just share 'me' instead. At least then the landscape would be familiar. These are uncharted waters – I may lose myself. High & low & inbetween. How many of me can there be? Both together? None at all? Who is who? Am I even me?"

Out of nowhere

"I was just listening to music + flicking thru my picture books. Thought all was OK. Sorta glad place was basically empty as still not really up to conversation + crowds but, still OK. Time passed. Then I realised I was swaying really hard back and forth + was scratching roughly + repeatedly at my upper arm. The skin was red and sore and I'd broken through leaving a sizeable raw patch. I hadn't even felt it. I told the nurse and she talked with me as she put a small dressing on it. I was quite worked up. If I'd been at home I'd have taken a tablet to calm myself down, but I couldn't here because they took them off me. I asked again and she finally got the doctor to sign off on a dose just before bedtime. They marked me down for small regular doses after that, but I didn't get today's because apparently I missed the 'meds call' – Stupid system."

Party

"I used to host really great parties – weekenders that would run from Friday night pizza to Sunday Breakfast. People would sleep when they felt the need and nip out for an hour or two if needed and come back... it was all so laid back and I loved it that way. I loved the full house, surrounded by friends. Back then almost everyone drank beer so we would spend time stacking the empties

into towers that could reach from floor to ceiling and stand under
their own pressure. A good party and we could sometimes make
two or three – it was our thing – and it was surprisingly fun. I miss
those parties. I miss the people."

The look

"It's so hard to talk about stuff, to ask for help, when you get the
look. (The look that says 'Here we go again, more of this miserable
moaning attention-seeking sh*t. I shouldn't have to listen to this.
She needs to get over herself already') It's so hard to keep talking
about stuff when no one really takes you seriously; they just
dismiss your pain with a casual euphemism and a swift change of
subject."

Blanket of the night

"As the blanket of night draped itself about the town, I once again
found myself walking the shadowy streets alone. I was striding on
with purpose, hood up and arms wrapped in tight against the cold: I
was trying to outrun something but I didn't know what. I was trying
to purge the overwhelming, suffocating thoughts and the pain they
gave birth to, yet they wafted behind me in a trail that I couldn't
shake off. I walked faster but they still found me. I had left the
house because the crushing intensity was made worse by being
closed in, being trapped; the night air was calling to me, offering a
balm to ease the unnamed turmoil. I needed to escape, to run,
from everything, everybody - I dove into the night without once
considering where I would end up because, most of all I was trying
to outrun myself. I wasn't thinking clearly because I was trying not
to think at all - I'd had enough and offered the pain up to the night.
Had my Hubby not come and brought me safely home, I don't know
how long I would have walked blindly into the darkness or where I
would have ended up. Sometimes, the voices cry louder as I walk,
but tonight I did manage to purge most of that which had sought to
overwhelm me. Tonight I nestled into a loving hug and welcomed
the emptiness, the ease of thought - my mind was my own again."

Give it your best shot

"The light shouted loudly from a chink in the curtains and its call
dragged me into a new day. Light? My head didn't even rise from
the pillow to pose the question; why was it light? A string of

expletives hung in the air like chorus to the song of rising panic. The phone was dead. The phone hadn't charged. The phone hadn't offered the promised alarm call. The phone nearly hit the wall.

But no, I wouldn't be distracted – I plugged in a different power cable and time stretched into agonising eternity while it processed the coded input. 10am. SH*T. Well it could have been worse. I made a hurried call to work and apologised then I flew around the upper floor of the house like a whirling dervish as I tried to get ready.

The roads were free of slippery frost and the journey into work surprisingly took a little less time than usual. Weary eyed but smiling, I stepped into the office and began to get everything switched on and ready. The day couldn't proceed without a cup of coffee so I quickly made one, only to find that the milk had soured and unwelcome bits of it were now floating in my cup. So, this is how the day is going to go is it? Well come on – give it all you've got! I'm in good form. I'm feeling good. It will take more than a temperamental smart phone and some soured milk to throw me off my stride. Come at me if you dare… but you'll have a fight on your hands…"

Eeyore and Tigger

"Today I feel..............
Scrambles around bin of crumbled paper scraps with mood suggestions
Well, I may as well just pick one at random because my emotional state defies definition right now - I genuinely am all over the place. No sooner have I identified one mood state and begun to address it, but I feel another rise up to supplant it. This afternoon alone, I have swung from intense depression to bouncing childlike excitement and happiness to intense anxiety to hypersensitivity and teasing paranoia to cruel distraction and extreme disinterest and back to thoroughly miserable again.

"Today I've been Eeyore and Tigger and I've been the blur as they run round and round the tree."

Right this minute, I would say the blur is persisting - Is it possible that I am entering a mixed episode? God, I really hope not because the last time I had one of those it was worse than the depression and I lived those days constantly on the edge of screaming. I've learnt how to begin to deal with the depression and the hypomania when they present independently but this rolled up,

mixed up, messed up pile of cr*p that is filling my head right now leaves me defenceless. I don't know what to do, or for that matter, what not to do. I only remember feeling like this once before - years ago - in the first year after diagnosis. I hated it then and I'm not feeling too enamoured tonight either. Is it a mixed episode? I don't have enough experience to know for sure, but really, what else could it be? I vaguely remember reading that mixed episodes only occur in bipolar I but even though I am bipolar II, it seems the only sensible explanation right now. Like I said - Eeyore, Tigger and a confusing blur of the two - Intensely happy and sad mixed together with fair measure of anxiety - shifting so often I can't get a handle on what's happening.
Feeling somewhat lost and helpless in the face of it all."

Step back

"I step back from aggression, avoid confrontation & regularly say nothing to maintain the status quo. I have become a deferential wimp."

On the edge

"Oh, what a transformational thing it is indeed to sit on the edge of a conversation; fully present yet without contributing more than a laugh or a smile. The interaction of others, the arising themes and unintended revelations - it's all quite compelling. Once or twice I thought to join them, to express an opinion, but truthfully, it was more beneficial to remain silent. Had they known I was the very thing maligned by their collective nattering, they may have spoken differently but I'd rather know the truth of things. I could have raised a lone voice against the tirade of disapproval but I remained instead on the edge of the conversation and listened."

Letterbox

"When I was first diagnosed, I was so worn down and weary that I accepted without question the medication prescribed for me; I was told it would work and there and then, that was all I cared about. We talked about it and I read the literature recommended to me so I felt reasonably prepared. I had even accepted the difficult truth that I could possibly be taking medication for the rest of my life. I was Okay with that. It only took a few weeks for noticeable changes to manifest and I was pleased to feel the shadow of my depressed and suicidal mood melt away. Well, what do you know? The meds are actually working! There was no wave of a magic wand – there was no overnight change – but little by little I began to find myself again. I felt hopeful.

About 8-12 months in however, I started to fight it – I kept taking the pills but I complained bitterly to myself as I did so – blaming the pills – blaming the professionals – feeling quite betrayed because in all those early discussions, I'd never once had a conversation that adequately addressed how I was feeling. I had desperately wanted rid of the depression but it wasn't until it was gone, that I fully understood what untreated hypomania really was. I ached with a nameless emptiness and began to wonder how this loss could possibly be reconciled. I had never attributed that boundless energy and racing creativity etc to an illness; I wanted it back – How dare the damn Lithium have stolen it! This is normal they said. They actually said it was exactly what was supposed to happen!! Intellectually I had known to expect it, but when it happened my very soul was fragmented and unrecognisable. I tried to talk about it but I just couldn't find the words; they just told me it was normal and smiled reassuringly. It's one of those 'had to be there' things – no book can adequately describe the desperation and panic experienced when bipolar meds start to reign things in. I was confused and desperate. I needed to be angry but didn't know where to direct it so it started to come back in on me.

I felt like I'd woken up in hospital bed after multiple leg fractures and been told "It's ok, we were able to treat it – you can be yourself again, walk all you like, there'll be no pain – it's just, well, you'll never run again – you'll never ride a bicycle -you'll never dance"

I should have been grateful that the Lithium had pulled the scope in, had given me a more peaceful place within myself in which to live. I shouldn't have blamed it for shutting out the exhilaration of life because it has taken the crushing despair with it. I should have been happy with the middle ground. It's a lot more than some people ever get. I wasn't happy though – I was miserable and angry. I came so very close to stopping taking the pills. If you were an adrenalin junkie – how happy would you be to be told "From now on you can't ride extreme roller coasters but hey, it's Okay because you can go on the drifting log flume all you like!" I know, I know – disbelief, shock, denial, and a sudden urge to smack the guy in the face and discontinue treatment.

That was all about five years ago – So – What did I do?

I trusted them and I stuck with it, and bit by bit I began to feel happier in my little letterbox world. I'd be lying if I said I never again longed for the rest of it but I can see now that when everything got pulled in for me, it just bought me closer to the experience of the general population. I can see that I'd been trying to live in a way that was not sustainable and it WAS nearly the death of me. The transition was difficult and emotional but now I don't blame Lithium for ruining my life – I thank it for saving me."

Dimmer switch

"Last night on Twitter, I promised I would write about my Friday – no matter how it played out; I was optimistic and was looking forward to today.
11.10am
Friday is 'sausage bap' day – I enjoyed my little treat – totally yummy. I'm at my desk now at break time and I have to say – so far this day isn't playing out so well – nothing has gone wrong, nothing is even out of routine, but since I got out of bed there has been a lingering shadow on my morning. I am not depressed. I am not upset. I am quietly uneasy. I have no clue how to adequately deal with such a subtle and intelligent foe: I feel it would take the very distillation of my breath, for that seems to be where it hides. I am slow in movement and laboured in thought. My mind searches for a hook to hang the feeling on, but all it can come up with is "exhausted" I am not tired. I am not even remotely tired, but as the explanation is apologetically offered I have no reasonable challenge. I seek to close my eyes and immerse myself in the emptiness - hoping that the air there would be pure, and the nameless parasite would wither and die. I seek to immerse myself in a silence so deep that even my enquiring spirit is still. My senses present a world I would rather avoid – it is just a little too loud, a little too bright, a little too much of everything. I seek to withdraw; I cannot. I sit uncomfortably at my desk instead – wishing the world about me had a dimmer switch.
3.01pm
I have managed to get some work done - not as much so far today as on a normal Friday though. That annoys me – I'm willing to do the stuff but progress is greatly inhibited by that vague nameless something that clings to me. It has made me so pre-occupied that I can't even think of IT in any clear terms. I can discern no reason for its presence and can formulate no strategy to combat it; a tiny seed of frustration now grows in its shade. I still feel slightly overwhelmed by life around me and long so badly to cradle into silence that it is beginning to ache. In a couple of hours I go

straight from my desk to an evening with family – it will kill me or cure me!"

Disgruntled

"A brand new bottle of little yellow pills sits quite disgruntled on the bedside cabinet, cast aside in favour of something much stronger. The smugness of the something stronger was soon eroded by the arrival of bottled beer. One way or another, her mind would find peace tonight; sleep may yet come. Tomorrow may yet be better."

Melancholy

"The cello softly plays and the air about me, heavy with melancholy, becomes easier to breathe. My tears brush my cheek with tenderness and I allow the unnamed sadness to wrap itself about me. It is familiar. It is comforting. I close my eyes and listen to the cello play - evocative, embracing. Smiles and tears nestle together into that rarest of moments."

A coping mechanism runs amuck

"When I am hypomanic (the high of my bipolar II spectrum) I have many of the common symptoms including impaired judgement and reckless behaviour. These manifest differently each time with one exception - I always have a problem with reckless spending - I know it happens - I try to guard against it where I can but still every single episode leaves a trail of bills I can ill afford to pay. Over the years I have managed to dial it back somewhat, buying smaller stuff or buying stuff that will at least to some degree be useful. Even with these plans in place my mixed episode caused a lot of damage. I bought an unneeded television upgrade at over half a month's wage, I ate out a lot more than usual, I bought gifts for other people, and on top of all that....looking at my bank statement now, 59% of my spending is attributed to unnecessary online shopping. I know it must be hard for others to understand why I let this happen; it just gets away from me and I either justify my purchases or live in denial until the episode fades and my bank statement arrives showing me where I need to focus to try and fix everything. You may think I am simply of weak character and to attribute this over-spending to my illness is a convenient lie; it is not. It is a real problem. It has been with me for years and it has been much much worse in the past. I am getting a little better at dealing with it each time but as you have seen, even with timely restrictions put in place it is an ongoing challenge; a coping mechanism runs amuck and in cruel metamorphosis mid-episode, becomes a compulsion. I am living with it all as best as I can."

I've said it before...

"I have said it before - I will say it again -
"Conversation is NOT the same as communication"
It is so sad to see these two constantly confused.
Conversation is an essential social tool. Worthwhile communication is a skill.
Skills are not finite - they demand commitment and development."

Elaine Fogarty

Random mood chart entries

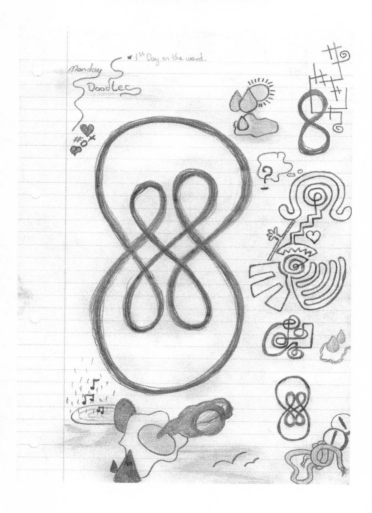

Elaine Fogarty

"Everything is going wrong – we have had frozen pipes, burst pipes, problems with the water supply, problems with the car not starting, and now major problems with electrical system. We've had no washing machine for ages now, the heat is off because of the burst pipe and we have no water and Hubby is ill with some rotten stomach bug and me? Well, I'm strangely calm about it all. I feel somewhat dethatched, like it's happening to someone else."

"Very upsetting! Dreamt I was out alone with the two boys and they both fell in the water. I can't really swim so was horrified. Decided to try and jump in to try and save them but when I looked they were far apart – could only get one – had to choose – managed to paddle over and get one to the bank. Someone arrived just at that moment and pulled him out but when I turned round the other was gone. Afterwards it still upset me a lot particularly that I'd made a choice. It was probably more a case of one was closer. Simple as – that but still – very upsetting."

"Last night was really bad. Horrible dreams – all about cutting myself badly, lots of blood. At one point I even cut my finger off which was weird. But the cutting images were so clear. I kept waking feeling really upset, and then I'd sleep, dream badly and wake again."

"Bad dreams last night. Spiralling downward. Feeling desperate. Needing some help. No one wanted to know. Tried person after person – ignored or turned away."

"Today was a tough day at work – it's so hard to cope at the minute. Staying on top of things – just! Withdrawn. Noticeably quieter. A lot slower.
Thinking about death and dying a lot. Last night was more of the same."

"Burnt the potatoes to the pan again – really badly, smoke everywhere and a thick burnt on pan layer. I just can't stay focussed when cooking. I've put stuff in the oven and not turned it on – stupid crap like that. Feel stupid and useless. Happens way too often – Getting really good at rescuing ruined pans though."

"Bad concentration – screwing up the money now – gave £60 instead of £40 in a shop and only got change of £40. Didn't realise until too late. Felt terrible."

"Difficult day in work. Trying to learn new stuff on the computer stock control system and getting very stressed out as finding it difficult to grasp. Feel so stupid. Too many variables to remember – felt actually sick and was panicky on the inside while trying to appear calm on the outside. Took a diazepam and it helped the panic but home now and still feeling sick. Annoyed – used to be able to take to new stuff so easily. They must think I am so stupid ☹"

"Teeth ache a little and I know it's because I've begun clenching my teeth all the time. Trying to stop it but it sort of happens without me realising most of the time. My dentist isn't at all happy about it."

"Very stressed overall as still clenching my teeth badly, still feeling sick most of the day and headachy and absolutely no focus/concentration. Money worries still very much in the back of my mind. All this stress not helping – although thankfully sleeping not too bad, I can feel myself getting very low. Thinking about cutting again today and I haven't done that in a while. Three weeks worth of ironing still waiting to be done and mess everywhere! Haven't filled my tablet box, haven't showered in a good while, and haven't brushed my teeth much, no clothes ironed ready for tomorrow – now out. And haven't had anything to eat since lunch yesterday and its now after 10pm. Mess and jobs needing done piling up everywhere. Need a hug. Can't afford to take any time off work so struggling through – SO difficult. Just want to sleep or at least curl up somewhere dark and quiet."

"Feel like crap – feeling snowed under. Stressed. Right now I feel queasy sick, my head is pounding and I have sore teeth from clenching them all the time. I'm restless yet I'm exhausted. Just so worried about everything and I'm scared it will only get worse."

"It's so great spending time with the whole family – everybody – all together; it sure is noisy but today I'm in a good place and it doesn't bother me. It reminds me that I do have lots of people around me and that I don't have to feel so alone. I know I should grab hold of moments like these – mundane made special by the smiles of family."

"Hanging in the split second just before the rollercoaster accelerates down the steep hill...know the drop is coming, know it's gonna be bad, but there's f**k all can be done about it. – Posted about it on facebook – no one even commented. Feel so alone. Hate this. It's coming. Last night I went to bed at 9.30 exhausted but couldn't get over to sleep. When finally did, woke at about 4 after an awful nightmare where I murdered someone – stabbed them multiple times – blood and screaming. Horrible. Had to take some meds to calm down enough to get back to sleep. Slept in later than usual this morning – awake but just couldn't get out of bed. Teeth hurt, stomach churning already and my face is still covered in spots – it's all stress. I know it is."

"Bah humbug – there is a very good chance my Christmas cards won't get written."

"Hair is greasy and sticking to my head and itching, I'm still wearing that favourite woolly sweater and I know I look like crap – thing is – I just don't care. I got out of bed didn't I, I managed a day at work didn't I, I'm so tired of pretending everything is alright. I just want to curl up somewhere quiet and dark and be alone."

"I did not need this. I know there is nothing I can do about it but it has just caused some switch in my head to flip. I've had enough. I've rung in sick for the charity work tomorrow and I'm heading to bed now. SO worried about how we will ever get out of this hole – I'd take off sick because I'm finding it hard to focus and cope with the constant thoughts and the nausea and the headaches and the teeth ache etc – but I can't afford to take off. Feel trapped in a corner. Rising panic. Can hardly breathe."

"I'm standing on the beach, just waiting for the Tsunami to hit."

"Had really bad scary dreams last night. Took ages this morning to settle. Still in my jammies and feeling sorry for myself – no energy or interest in doing anything. Work is getting harder and I'm dreading going in tomorrow. I'm on my own right now and can't stop thinking about cutting – it always makes things better."

"Something made me think about it. I haven't washed my hair since the 2nd (10 days) and I've been wearing virtually the same clothes every day since the 6th (7 days) I've been feeling so bad I didn't care, it was a miracle I got up and out at all let alone worry about stuff like that. But how did it go on so long and I'm only noticing now? How did it go on so long without Hubby noticing? Or did he notice and ignored it – which is worse. Others must have noticed? – don't know. I will drag myself to the shower this evening and make an effort. Really don't feel like it."

"Feeling very positive today, particularly after my psych appointment. Coping very well in work at the moment – just working slowly and systematically. I think joining Twitter has really helped boost my mood as I don't feel so isolated anymore and I can discuss or vent with people who share the same issues."

"I didn't sleep well at all. I woke feeling really restless. I'm just so pre-occupied. Worried that I've ruined everything; I didn't mean to scare them but I can't undo it. I have no one to talk to... I am off on paid leave, alone in the house and incredibly anxious. I'm very vulnerable right now, overwhelmed, confused – so very isolated. I shouldn't be alone right now. I meditated and calmed a little. Also spoke to CPN. Almost keen now to see tomorrow; to draw a line under this mess and move on."

"Saw every half hour in bed last night and when I did sleep I dreamt of cutting, I woke and I thought about cutting. By the time morning came I wanted to cut. I almost did, I still have my blade in my bag. Instead I took a dark red biro and drew the lines on my arm. I went to work and when I thought about cutting I'd look at the lines and pretend they were real. It wasn't as good as the real thing but I'm told I should try it. I still want to cut. Damn."

"I'm not stupid. I enjoy watching Brian Cox or Stephen Hawking talk about the nature of the universe, time travel and the nothingness of matter. I enjoy tossing around classic philosophical questions. I can even line all the shopping up properly in batches on the belt so it packs easily into waiting bags. Why then, can I not understand simple instructions on operating a new computer database system? I may not be stupid but I sure as hell feel stupid."

"We went to see a film. The upper level was pretty crowded because the screen hadn't opened yet. Hubby had to leave me to go buy some 3D glasses. While he was away, they removed the barrier and everyone surged forward at once. Passed me, from behind, beside. There were so many and so, so close. I felt scared and began to take a panic attack right there in front of people. Why did I have to draw attention? – that made it worse. Luckily, just then Hubby came back. I was ok inside the theatre – I settled – as everyone was in their assigned seats. I can cope with crowds better if they are seated – it feels more controlled."

"I don't feel depressed. But I don't feel quite normal either. Hell, what is normal anyway? I feel... detached... like everything is happening around me and to me, but doesn't really involve me at all. I'm sort of seeing life all float by me. I'm sort of not in it – but I am. I can't explain it."

"Thinking through the details of my suicide plan but not emotionally ready to use it.
It's all still thoughts."

"Been thinking today about the appointment I had with that CBT guy. Don't recall much of the specifics of what he said but I do remember the 100 Acre Wood story. It has stuck in my head and even though it's a simple story, I've found it useful – to help me remember it I've bought a Pooh and Piglet keying on eBay. Gotta love the simplicity."

"Somewhere in and around Valentine's Day I started a Twitter account and I'm getting addicted. I'm finally able to speak my mind, to share with people who truly understand as they are going through the same thing. I even spent an hour late last night in dm to a young girl who was in real despair and she seemed to find our conversation helpful. I don't feel quite so alone any more. This Twitter may be the best thing I did to help myself in a long time."

"Spent two days at home in bed feeling really sorry for my self – a rather rapid onset of depression. It floored me. But tried using my CBT training and although not 100%, I was back in work a couple of days later. This is exactly what I was hoping the therapy could help with – to nip things in the bud before they get really bad."

"Hypomania? Wide awake and up before 5am on a bl**dy Saturday – and tidying and organising into the bargain! I had been optimistic and set an alarm for 9am."

"That medication has got to go! Its effects on mood and sleep have been great, the best I've felt in a long time, BUT the side effect of dry mouth just will not settle; in fact it has gotten worse. Constant and irritating, there's swelling which is uncomfortable and leads to me biting the sides of my tongue which then goes to little sores. The tip and back of the tongue are 'raw' and these past two nights I've been woke by the discomfort. This morning I had to peel my tongue off the roof of my mouth – ouch! I will not put up with this."

"Hypomania project – I finished my 'smile box' tonight. A little wooden chest with gathered keepsakes – such a good idea – don't know why I didn't do it sooner."

"Things got on top of me today and I stupidly cut in work. – REALLY Stupid!!!"

"Today a child asked me if I was going to have a baby! I tried to hide it, but I was really upset. I know I've put on an awful lot of weight since I went on that new meds – have gained back the whole stone I lost last year. Of course the kid was young and didn't understand why I was upset. Could cry."

"Crashing after a three-week hypomanic episode – exhausted, drained, empty and p*ssed off – Mad at the world, mad at myself, mad at the illness. Want the high back."

"Everything's getting a bit difficult. I go over it all over and over again and it seems so hopeless. I feel useless. How come everyone round me is doing so well? Feel so weary and disinterested. Christmas is coming and everyone else is getting excited – I'm dreading it. My routine is already thrown way off and I'm faced with that horrible deadline and all the expectation that is loaded into it. Everyone else seems to be loving it – I'm beginning to dread it. ~ It's overwhelming. I hate all the noise and really hate the crowds and hate that I just don't have the money to do it all right. I hate that I'm incapable of hosting a proper family Christmas. I'm just so useless. I JUST WANT TO BE ALONE. For everyone else's sake I'll try to enjoy Christmas but already I'm feeling depressed and no one seems to care."

"Hair needs washing but I can't be bothered showering. Haven't even brushed my teeth in a few days. Wish I didn't have to get up at all, wish I didn't have to go in to work. I wish I didn't have to keep trying to pretend nothing is wrong. It's all so exhausting. I look like crap – folk in work think I have a cold. I wish it was a cold."

"Just lay in bed till late afternoon because Colin was away out from early morning and I just didn't see the point in getting up – I wouldn't have if he hadn't rung I don't think. When I got up I checked Facebook when I checking my email and was very upset no one had commented on or contacted me about my last 2 status posts. Surely those who know me and my condition would have seen from that that I was really struggling? Does no one care? Been thinking a lot about cutting and suicide by cutting – been thinking through all the details. Sounds bad I know but planning it all out in my head made me feel better. As for the cutting, well, I've been using my shoulder lately – small cuts, easily covered and hidden. This has been like a mini little breakdown – something just snapped on Friday afternoon when I got that message – it was one bit of bad news too many. I've shut down, I hardly talk, I'm not eating, and I spend most of my time in bed or in a curl up ball on the sofa hugging a small cushion. I'm not sure I've been taking my meds right. I can't remember. Not sure if they help anymore. Right now I don't care. Either not sleeping or sleeping way too much. I'm a mess. Hubby is actually so worried he thought I should ring and see if I could get into the ward for a few days! I told him they wouldn't do it."

"My mood hasn't improved, but I'm pretty sure it has now bottomed out – I feel strangely calm. Still having the urge to self harm to silence dark thoughts but my butterfly is still there and I don't want to kill it."

"What a change from yesterday – today work was slow and tedious. I just haven't felt right since I got up this morning. I can't describe it – weird. Mild headache, somewhat distracted and disinterested. Just plodding through the day until I could get home and just lie up in front of the telly – not that it's much more than noise at the minute because I really don't care to properly watch anything. Today my mood is sort of empty and I just sort of let the world wash over me and try not to get involved. A few days ago I felt fine, actually very good, and even a little high, now everything is so different. Don't know what is going on."

"Suicidal – alone – had planned, prepared and was minutes from implementing the plan. Talked myself down, then shaken/scared by how close I had come."

"There have been a lot of negative posts here lately but it's not all doom and gloom – today was actually a very good day."

"Still thinking about the whole 'suicidal' thing – was convinced that being totally open with everyone was the best idea – now really doubting that. Are raging flames and poisonous smoke outside the door any less real just because you take your hand off the handle and escape through the window instead? – Everyone, bar one, that I have shared the story of that night with, has reacted by playing it down and pretending it wasn't real. I know it was real. There's a pile of stuff lying in a hedge somewhere now because I managed to talk myself out of it. I know how close I came to using that stuff –
I've stopped trying to convince people. It only makes me feel worse. I've been told I over analyse, that I place everything under a magnifying glass and try to understand it. Maybe so – but if I hadn't been able to think like that, to understand like that, I wouldn't have been able to use my CBT skills and talk myself down. It was as real and as close as I've come in about six years and no one will believe me.
So – that proves there is no point in sharing the truth with the real world."

"Settling into work again well – actually enjoying it. Mood stable again except for some anxiety. Fighting the urge to cut again – scratching instead which is a marginal improvement... things do seem to be getting better. I actually would dare to use the word stable"

"Anxiety enveloping me, depression stalking me and the stench of loneliness hangs heavy in the air. Waves of nausea and panic carry me through the day till I come to rest, trapped in the very corner of hopelessness, tasting the saltiness of uncontrollable tears. Depression lurks in the shadows and whispers to me, telling tales of things to come, and that scares me. I wish it all to go away and were my wishes like drops of rain, they still could not nourish the seed of hope. –
Posted this on Facebook and no one commented, let alone contacted me. No one cares. Tough day in work – really distracted. Couldn't concentrate properly – felt like someone was shouting in my ear all day – so hard to get any work done."

"I'm glancing through some old sheets and it all seems doom and gloom – I do have lots of good days – must have just never got round to writing those days."

"Bizarrely, feeling a little bit better today is making things worse. I'm not quite well enough to be up and stuck in, making full use of a day. Off work but I am well enough now to notice the passage of time and to get REALLY bored. I don't know what to do. I did pull together the motivation to bake a cake but that was about it – quite proud of myself on that one. I hate being in the house alone all day, and a late day at that because Hubby is driving today. Definitely going back to work on Monday. My mood is lifting and even if the concentration is crap I can just go slowly."

"Really restless and fidgety. There's so much going on in my head I can't concentrate on anything – I know I can be a little like this most of the time but this is worse than usual, not even watching TV. I can't seem to settle. Want to crawl into bed in a nice quiet dark room and get away from it all."

"I did it again – I was out walking the country roads alone in the middle of the night. Hubby noticed I was gone and drove around for a while until he found me and brought me home. Neither of us knows how long I was out there, but I'd covered a sizable distance. It was cold and raining too, yet I hadn't really noticed. I've been really depressed of late and the thoughts were becoming very oppressive; I needed room to be able to think I guess but I can't even remember exactly what I was thinking about. It wasn't fluffy kittens and summer picnics that's for sure. Dark thoughts for a dark night."

"I'd never drive the car deliberately off the road... other people could get hurt... my problems aren't their problems. I'd never do that... Why would they ask?"

"Lithium – Quietiapine – At last a cocktail that seems to be working. Of course I still have my benzos, but they're not for consistent use. No – this is it for the foreseeable and, some manageable dry mouth aside, I'm pleased with how it's doing its job. Most notably, I feel mellow. Yes, that's it, loving that word – mellow – without feeling dazed as I had on other meds. The first couple of months were hard to deal with because of the super-sedative effect but once the meds bedded in all that just melted away and I'm left with the ability to sleep so much better too (which is a great bonus.) Still using the little daily box meds case that I got after the home crisis team hauled me over the coals for non-compliance; it's easier now – the box sits out on the bench next to the fridge – I can't miss it. Overall, I'd have to say I'm happy with my meds – we're getting along great. Long may it continue!"

"I used to burn candles all the time, had them all over the place including the hearth of the open fire. I also used to wear long lightweight hippy style full skirts. It doesn't take genius to see where this is going – I kept forgetting about them – three times I nearly set my skirt on fire and I've gone to bed many times and left them burning. You'd think a grown adult would know better! I don't mind being forgetful or unobservant (everyone is like that from time to time), but it was starting to get dangerous so the lighting of candles has been greatly curtailed; I miss them. The yoga teacher in me still wants to sit in a room lit only by candlelight but I've got to be sensible. This is the sort of small stuff that other people laugh off; I try to, but it's not just about candles and skirts – I know that."

"Hypomania is a kaleidoscope that complicates my day, yet somehow still manages to make me feel good."

"I'm so terribly stressed and I can't seem to do anything about it. Nothing is working. I'm just getting more and more wound up as the days tick by. I'm maybe too far in to be able to see a way out. This sucks. ...Stress – a real buzz word I know – but it's buzzing for a reason – it's incredibly dangerous. Give it an exoskeleton and some slathering menacing jaws and it could have its own sci-fi film. Stress will stalk you, tease you from the safety of others and then run you until you are completely exhausted. It is vicious. It is relentless. It will haunt your dreams and shadow your day. It will not stop. Stress is an ugly son of a b*tch whose only mission is to devour you. 'Oh a little stress is actually good for you.' That's B*ll*ocks! Stress is trying to kill me and I'm sure as hell not gonna hang around to see how he finally manages it. I'm going to run, and run hard. Maybe he'll tire first?"

"If I google the online me, I'm top of the first page. If I google the real me, It's like standing in a hall of mirrors – I can't see myself for all the other mes. Does that mean something? Should it mean something? Does it matter? Do I really need to know why? Does it mean that one identity is more important or even more real than the other? Oh, here we go again – the nature of duality and the quest for identity... the subject that just never goes away. Google, you've got a lot to answer for... Now I'll never get any sleep."

"Ever noticed how, when a cat yawns, infinity pours out of their mouth and the jaws open so very wide, it looks for a moment, like they're going to keep going, turn in on themselves, and the cat will swallow its own head? I wish I were skilled in computer graphics and then I could make it happen – that would be so cool. Surreal, but cool. It always makes me smile – surreal is just so me."

"Sometimes I can get quite aggressive, verbally that is, not physically – but still, it hits so quick I'm not really aware until it's almost over, 'til I start to calm down. I can see how some would find that intimidating or even threatening so I worry a lot about it maybe happening when I'm among strangers – I could end up putting myself at risk if those strangers saw me as a threat. That's another one of the reasons that I don't like going out alone. I can't control stuff like that and it could bite me in the ass so easily. It doesn't happen often but it's still a risk factor."

"Did I ever mention that the film *It's a Wonderful Life* is quite possibly the best therapy for a weary and despairing mind?"

"Someday I'll maybe figure out what's going on – but for now – I'll settle for just coping the best I can. That's all anyone could do. That's all I should be doing – it's time to stop swimming against the current."

Selected quotes

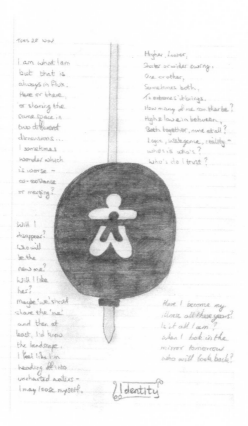

Tues 28 Nov

I am what I am
but that is
always in flux.
Here or there,
or sharing the
same space in
two different
dimensions...
I sometimes
wonder which
is worse –
co-existance
or merging?

Will I
disappear?
Who will
be the
new me?
Will I like
her?
Maybe 'we' should
share the 'me'
and then at
least, I'd know
the landscape.
I feel like I'm
heading into
uncharted waters –
I may loose myself.

Higher, Lower,
Shorter or wider swing.
One or other,
Sometimes both,
To extremes it brings.
How many of me can there be?
High & low in between,
Both together, none at all?
Logic, intelligence, reality –
who is is who's?
Who's do I trust?

Have I become my
illness all these years?
Is it all I am?
when I look in the
mirror tomorrow
who will look back?

Identity

Elaine Fogarty

The following are original 'quotes' from my own work.

~ ~ ~ ~

"Trust not what I present to you as truth, but rather stand upon it and look to the horizon, there to find your own."

"When you feel as delicate as a floating bubble, everything and everyone around you starts to look an awful lot like a pin."

"I would scarce have strength to walk this earth, were it not for God's grace pushing gently back with encouragement, every step I take."

"Depression is like struggling through 3ft snowdrifts. Suicidal thoughts can hit like an avalanche or hide in the falling flakes."

"I hope your day never sees the rain, but at least you now know which tree to shelter under."

"There is little more cruel in life, than to be, at heart, a 'social animal' yet find yourself cursed with social anxiety."

"Above all else, be kind. You never know the burdens other people carry."

"The meds take the edge off – the rest is just life."

"Over-thinking hasn't killed me yet; it keeps the demons distracted."

"Mindfulness is just falling awake – everyone should try it."

"I enjoy reading philosophy – *Winnie the Pooh* is my favourite text"

"Political correctness is mankind gone crazy. I mean womankind, no personkind, no citizens of the earth, no – oh, you see what I mean?"

"When drawn from the shadows, ignorance withers under the sun."

"Hypomania is like surfing – you know that eventually you're going to crash but, while you find yourself up there, you may as well ride the wave and enjoy yourself."

"To conquer an enemy you must first name him, then, with steeled purpose, attack with knowledge of his very soul."

"Consuming darkness is but a veil drawn over bless'd light and hope."

"To walk slowly in the rain is to feel God's hand wipe away a tear."

"Reality is born of perception; the challenge of life is to manage that perception."

"Conversation is not communication: people need to learn the difference."

"A hug is the single greatest therapeutic tool available."

"You haven't lived until warm sand has squished up through your bare toes as you walked, or dew-laden grass brushed the soles of your feet."

"Perhaps God messed up my brain chemistry just so I could actually see the lost reality of his world."

"As the faeries dance in fading moonlight, so too does my soul embrace the coming darkness"

"Gratitude can lift us above all troubles, for in realising our blessings we transcend entitlement, and look instead to how we may help others."

"Stillness of breath will guide you, not where you want to go, but where you need to go."

"When depression stares back from the mirror, cling tightly to your true self."

"Nothing said, good or bad, is ever lost; words hang invisible about us."

"Bipolar disorder is not a curse; it is merely the vehicle by which I explore my existence."

"I've learnt a lot from my computer. Sometimes I need to shut down and reboot too."

"Self esteem decreases exponentially in the presence of dismissal and betrayal."

"To remember what one never knew, is to find true peace."

"Conformity is OK in small doses."

"Many can speak their mind, but few can speak their spirit. It is laudable indeed to be able to articulate the nature of one's true self."

"A strange comfort exudes from misery – happiness is too big a risk."

"If my own thoughts conspire against me, how should I then proceed, but with faith?"

"How refreshing it would be, should everyone at once throw down their mask and dare to leave the play behind."

"Life is binary – it really is that simple."

"The laughter of children is a balm to heal many a wound."

"Hope is an unshakeable belief in possibilities; nothing is inevitable."

"The internet is not a beast than needs tamed; it is a bird that teaches us how to soar."

"A perception filter is the means by which we experience life; immutable yet, simultaneously inviting change."

"Re-creating yourself to fill the mould of a diagnosis is as futile as trying to breathe under water."

"I'd rather you spoke the truth with a tear than lie to me with a smile."

"Dreams should never be feared; in fact, the lack of them can cripple a life."

"Poetry is like life – it works best when you just let it flow."

"I live a lot of my life in hindsight, because that's sometimes the only place where it makes sense."

"Sharing conversation is wonderful but sharing silence can sometimes achieve more."

"My life would have been pretty boring if I hadn't been bipolar; that's the thing about rollercoasters – they scare you near to death just to make you feel alive."

"Once you engage with the moment, time itself slows to help you get better acquainted."

"Open the lid of a keepsake box and all the best bits of your life are there to greet you; ten minutes with that box is like an hour's therapy."

"Self pity is like quicksand, for it will mercilessly pull you under and claim your life."

"From the birth of steam power man has known the importance of release valves, yet we continue to ignore our own. Whether arrogance or folly, it will be the end of us."

"God created geodes to teach us the importance of looking past appearances."

Elaine Fogarty

Bipolar disorder Q &A

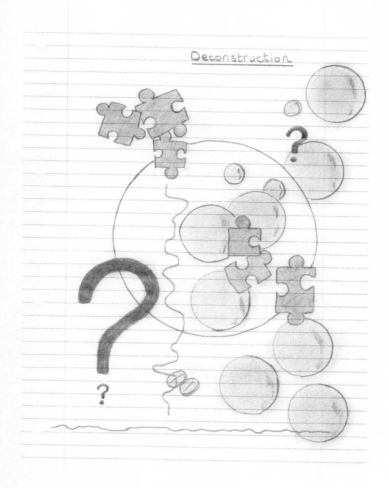

Elaine Fogarty

I should again point out that I am not a Mental Health Professional. These answers reflect only my own experience and opinion.

So, what is it?

Put as simply as I can, bipolar is a mood disorder that causes extended and intense mood swings (episodes) beyond the 'norm' of the general population. There are periods of depression and mania (or hypomania). In some cases it is also possible to experience a mixed episode where both elements are present. Diagnosis further differentiates and refers to four main types – Bipolar I, Bipolar II, Cyclothymia and Rapid cycling. Bipolar I – a person has cycling periods of mania and periods of deep depression; in many cases the mania is dominant by timescale, but it may just be that it is more intense. Bipolar II – both depression and hypomania (a less intense form of mania) are present, but it is usually depression that dominates the mood cycle. Cyclothymia – a similar range within the mood cycle, but the episodes are less intense; I was told that this can develop into 'full' bipolar. Rapid cycling – a person falls into the category of bipolar I or II, but experiences four or more distinct episodes in a year. I refer to the period between episodes as stable rather than normal because a trace of the mood challenges often remains.

What is the difference between bipolar disorder and manic depression?

None. Manic depression was the name previously in common use. They are interchangeable.

Isn't that just the latest 'trendy' diagnosis?

There does seem to be a lot celebrities disclosing their illness lately... it would be easy to be cynical. It could be that the diagnosis percentages are the same as in 'our' world but that celebrities feel better able to raise the issue. It could of course be that they identify with the symptoms and report themselves as bipolar because it feels right; and yes, perhaps there are a few who like to add interest to their public image. I prefer to see the good in people, so if a celebrity discloses their bipolar, I applaud their strength and hope that they can find a way to use their status to raise awareness and address stigma.

Is there a cure?

Not yet – but the mechanisms of brain function in relation to bipolar are being studied; just as research found ways of managing the illness with medication, so it may yet discover a way to permanently address the issue. There is a growing movement of people who report to have cured their bipolar disorder by holistic means. The final answer will most likely draw on the experience of both fields.

You take lithium for that, right? Isn't it dangerous?

Lithium is extremely effective in treating bipolar, but it can be dangerous, even fatal in overdose; regular blood tests are essential while taking the medication to ensure levels do not become toxic. The blood tests are weekly or fortnightly at first, then settle into a three-month cycle. When taking this, it is important to manage fluid levels – anything that significantly disrupts the levels also alters the concentration of lithium.

Have you ever been locked up?

I assume you mean sectioned – no. Just before my diagnosis I went voluntarily on to a psychiatric ward for assessment: it was supposed to be for just three days, but stretched into four weeks. Once in, it didn't feel so voluntary, and I had to get passes to get out for a day or a weekend – stuff like that. Could I have just walked out the door before discharge? I honestly don't know that they would have let me. That doesn't bother me though, because deep down, I knew I needed help.

Ever try to kill yourself?

Try – no. Find myself sitting in the right place with everything I needed around me and thinking out the final pros and cons, trying to gather the courage to follow through – yes. At the time of writing this I am in my 40s and I have been in that place five times in my life.

Do you hide your mental illness?

I used to. I was afraid and embarrassed. I don't any more. It wasn't a decision I took lightly. If people ask, I answer. If I need help I ask for it. I discuss my experiences so that people can better understand what it is to be mentally ill. I'm done hiding.

How did you react to your diagnosis?

I was relieved. I'd been fighting the demons for most of my life and I hadn't understood what was happening, why it kept on happening or why indeed me at all. My diagnosis answered the questions for me and offered promise of treatment. I was overwhelmed by all the stuff being thrown at me at once and it took a while to let it sink in and adjust but I was happy about it. Relieved and happy.

Do all those meds not give you a load of side effects?

Most medication has side effects – some are barely noticeable and others in extreme can be quite distressing. It's different for each person and can even change over time for a long-term user. It is a trade-off. It has been six years from my diagnosis and first treatment plan and I've tried different things to end up where I am now; nothing is perfect but what I'm using now seems to be a good compromise. Some of the side effects I've experienced are: headaches, restless legs, severe dry mouth, manageable dry mouth, leaking from the breasts, clenching teeth, extreme drowsiness, severe weight gain, hand tremor, closing in of the throat, craving salt, feeling 'zombified', nausea, metallic taste in the mouth, jaundice and loss of sex drive. Not all at once of course and not all from the same meds.

Can you still cope at work?

I won't lie – work is incredibly difficult for me. I have ongoing issues like poor concentration, anxiety, pre-occupation, obsessive orderliness and persistent tiredness. I do very well though in my current post because they know about my mental illness and are very willing to offer support; I've been there just under 10 years now. I have, however, up until then had a patchy work history, most of the jobs were only two years or so (just enough time to have a major episode and become unable to function). Back then I didn't understand why I couldn't hold down a job but with hindsight, it was definitely the bipolar.

How common is bipolar disorder?

It affects men and women equally and most commonly presents mid-teens to thirties. The last figures I heard, affected population was placed at approximately 1%.

Does it affect your friendships?

Short answer: yes. I have social anxiety so 'getting out there' is difficult. Some I lost because my bipolar self did stupid stuff to ruin things. Some I lost in the wake of a mental ill health diagnosis – I think it scared them. I struggle to hold on to those I have left but I can let time slip by so much when I'm wrapped up in one of my episodes – often it is they who must make the first move and suggest getting together. It's hard for them because they have to cope with my mood swings, too. The trick is... not to dwell on the losses but focus instead on the remaining friendships.

Is there an 'upside' to bipolar?

I love the hypomania. When I'm high I feel like Me+. I have bags of energy, my confidence sky-rockets, and my brain runs super fast and figures out all the stuff I'd been struggling with. I get loads done, including many of the little unfinished projects. I write better and I'm much more creative. I like hypomania because I glide over life without actually having to get bogged down in the details. It just feels good, feels right. Thing is though, the crash when the episode finally ends REALLY sucks. I also love that my bipolar has made me much empathetic and it has made me a really good listener. I like that, because of the bipolar, I look for the good in people and I recognise that there are better ways to spent time than arguing and posturing. I'm convinced it has given me a different perspective on life and made me more creative. The despair I experience holds up in contrast to the world around me and lets me see the joy and beauty of it. I've made a lot of friends online too, because we share the same challenges – I'm blessed to be able to have people out there who totally understand.

I've seen BPD on social network sites – is this bipolar?

No, it's a common confusion – BPD actually stands for borderline personality disorder, which incidentally has much in common with bipolar.

When did you first realise you had it?

Until my diagnosis about six years ago, I'd never heard of bipolar disorder. I presented at the doctor's office in the wake of a near suicide; I'd struggled with depression most of my life and had just had enough! When the psychiatrist gave me the diagnosis the pieces immediately fell into place and all that scary and confusing stuff of years gone by just made sense.

Do you resent having bipolar?

No – I'm at a place now where I understand. Bipolar has been with me all my life, it has contributed so much (good and bad) and it has made me who I am today. When I sometimes look at the lives of others and feel cheated, I remind myself that they have their own issues to deal with; perhaps I am lucky to only have my mental illness. My experience with bipolar also means that I have been blessed with an opportunity to speak to others who are suffering or in crisis and let them know they are not alone. I accept it now.

I've heard you bipolars are all creative types. Is that true?

I can only speak for myself, but I do genuinely believe that there is a link between creativity and the bipolar mind.

Did you think much about mental illness before diagnosis?

No, not at all – I was vaguely aware of depression and I'd heard of schizophrenia and ADHD but didn't know any details. I bought into the whole 'crazies and padded cells' idea – I didn't think about it being all around me in people I knew.

What do you say to the people who claim bipolar disorder isn't real?

I respect their right to say it, but really, the only answer is, "Walk a mile in my shoes and feel the blisters for yourself!"

Does relaxation stuff help with bipolar?

Stress, agitation, inability to sleep, anxiety issues, rapid thoughts, headaches, teeth clenching, dark thoughts....... All these things and more can be helped by relaxation techniques; invaluable to a bipolar sufferer. The thing is, even though I am a qualified yoga teacher, even though I am a qualified relaxation therapist, even though my key-workers have offered much advice on how to use relaxation, I often find that it is incredibly difficult. It helps, but it takes work.

How long did it take you to learn how to spell psychiatrist?

Oh, not long – truthfully, about 5 years! Still get it wrong now and then.

Does a full moon really make the symptoms worse?

Wow, I've talked to a lot of people, I've read a lot of stuff, but I have never come across this idea before. I don't know. Some say young children and animals have a kind of sixth sense – maybe it's also true of those touched by madness? It's an intriguing idea and I'm way too open-minded to rule it out.

Do you still listen to music when depressed?

Not very much, but when I do I'm very fond of stuff like Metallica's 'Fade to Black.' When stable, my taste is much more eclectic.

Have you encountered stigma?

The one thing that continues to hurt is the barely unperceivable way in which people 'pull back' when you tell them you have a mental illness. I've also had people cross the room or stop to tie a pretend shoe lace just so they can avoid talking to me. They are frightened or repulsed or think it to be contagious – I don't know, but it is hard experience. It also bugs me when people assume the illness come with a serious drop in IQ – they can be really patronising sometimes.

Was school difficult with bipolar?

Again, going through school I didn't know it was bipolar. I had concentration issues, I had a fair measure of anxiety and I suffered even then from incredible depression. My school reports for primary school read very well – I was active in class and performing well. Round about the time I moved to my next school I started to get the waves of depression and my reports were peppered with statements like 'Could do so much better,' 'Doesn't participate,' 'Simply not trying,' 'When she applies herself...'
I did ok. I had some friends, joined some clubs. I was even a prefect, so I coped some of the time. I went as far as completing A-level stage and then, apart from some night classes and correspondence courses, I was done with schoolwork for ever. At 13 I was depressed, but at 13 I didn't understand the implications of that.

Have you ever told someone about your illness and then regretted it?

Yes, but this kind of thing happens to everybody at some stage doesn't it? – Such is life. It would be easy to let such things eat at me, but I really shouldn't.

How long did it take to get a diagnosis?

When I first started going to the doctor's, all I complained about was the depression so it was understandable that's what the dx was. I had been ill since childhood, accepted the depression diagnosis for years, and then back in 2006 I was so bad I ended up on a psychiatric ward for observation. That finally got me my correct diagnosis so in all, about 30 years. You may be shocked at that but it happens all the time. Thing is, we bipolars are so busy enjoying the highs that we don't see them as a problem, don't discuss them with the doctor, and in the absence of such important information, the doctors continue to misdiagnose. Bipolar is a bit like a little lizard sitting on a branch pretending to be a leaf – we are unlikely to see it because we aren't looking for it.

What's with the butterfly?

It's a temporary tattoo – it's there to dissuade me from self-harming. The idea comes from 'the butterfly project' and is very simple – place the tattoo or draw a butterfly on an area where you would usually self-harm.....try not to self-harm while the butterfly remains intact (this could be 1-5 days depending on how shower proof it is) It is an excellent coping strategy and, although originally aimed at teenagers, it works very well for a gal in her 40's.

Does CBT help?

Cognitive behavioural therapy won't work well for everyone, but it has become daily tool for me. I think it its really good. As time goes on you get better at it and it becomes so much easier to challenge the negative thoughts. I can honestly say that my CBT skills saved my life – they talked me down during my last near-suicide.

Those cuts on your arm... is that because of the bipolar?

Yes. Well, more specifically it's a coping mechanism that developed to deal with it. Somewhere along the line, my brain made a connection between self harm and feeling better. It must sound bad to someone who doesn't do it, but it is as real to me as the air I breathe – cuts, burns, scratches, scars, they all act as a release valve. We all know what happens to a pressure container when the release valve fails – my cuts keep me safe.

Is bipolar hereditary?

Most people believe that there is indeed a genetic pre-disposition toward bipolar disorder.

If it affects your thinking, can you still drive?

The illness itself can render a person unable to drive and certain medications can make it dangerous due to the strong sedative effect. In my case – following diagnosis I wasn't allowed to drive for nearly a year. When I did get my license back it was for three years only (some people never drive again and some only get one-year licences) Each renewal, information on my situation is requested from my doctor and the authorities can revoke a driving licence at any time if they deem you to be a danger to yourself or others. I do drive but only necessary and familiar journeys now – I don't do motorways and I don't like passengers. If I didn't need the car to get to work, I'd give up the driving all together; for me it's really difficult.

Is there an aspect of your illness that you try to play down?

Yes (well not play down as such, but avoid talking about): suicide. People get scared, flustered or angry – it's rarely worth it. I don't want to make people feel bad so most of the time I just keep it all to myself. I can talk to professionals about it but very few other people.

Are you hopeful for the future?

Right now, yes. The problem is that the future is not set.

What's a CPN?

It means Community Psychiatric Nurse. I was assigned one when I left hospital following my diagnosis and have been in regular contact ever since. A CPN can offer specialised advice on mental health and prove an excellent sounding board when unwell.

Does bipolar disorder make you hard to live with?

Actually, I'd have to be honest and say yes – at times. The mood swings can be unpredictable and frustrating for both of us and they can interfere with plans and social situations sometimes. When unwell I can get loud and angry and over-sensitive with little or no warning, or withdraw into a world of my own, maybe even 'shut down' completely for a while. When high I've got more energy than Lee Evans and advance to another whole level of multi-tasking. It's hard for people to keep up. I can sometimes spend money recklessly and I always seem to start into little 'projects' that become all-consuming. When hypomanic, I can be shifting furniture or spring cleaning when the world is asleep and when depressed, I generally try to ignore all housework out of existence. On a practical level we get by just fine, but poor Hubby constantly worries that he will say or do the wrong thing and make a situation worse for me, or even miss some really subtle but crucial warning sign that I am shifting into crisis. It's not all about my illness, but it is there and we have, over the years, worked out how to cope as a couple when it interjects. We're together 28½ years, so don't get me wrong, we've managed well. We've figured out the essentials of marriage; I put the toilet rolls on to the holder in the bathroom and he tops up the water in the filter jug in the fridge – once we figured stuff like that out, the rest was easy. And the bipolar? Well, we think it's all down to education – people with bipolar partners need to learn as much about the illness as possible.

Sorry, what's hypomania again?

Hypo means less than – so hypomania is the bipolar state similar to but less intense than mania. It is the 'high' of the bipolar II spectrum.

How do I know you won't do that [terrible behaviour] again?

Well, sadly, you can't. You can't because I can't. It's impossible to make a promise about something you have no control over. I will try my best not to do it but ultimately I may fail.

Has it ruined your life?

No – It has almost ended it a couple of times, but the world I cling to is still a good place. I have my challenges but most of the time I cope – I have a lot to be thankful for – life can be good.

How do you explain it to kids?

I keep it simple... I have this illness and sometimes it can make me feel very, very sad and sometime it can make me really, really happy and excited. It's nothing to be scared about. It's just an illness. It's no one's fault. You didn't do anything wrong to make it happen. I'll be ok. Is there anything you'd like to ask?

Do you say you HAVE bipolar or that you ARE bipolar?

Some people get very upset about a wrong choice here, but I'm going to have to be controversial and go with AM. You see, my bipolar has directly contributed to who I am today. It informs my perception and my perception creates my reality. I am living in a body, a mindset and a life that it helped to forge therefore I AM bipolar.

Would you flip the switch?

No, that would be unconscionable – If there were a switch placed in front of me now with the promise of one flip magicking away my bipolar disorder as if it had never happened, I couldn't do it – it would mean denying a big part of myself.

How do you cope with it?

In no particular order, some of my coping strategies are: spending time with family and friends, walking, CBT, going for long drives, meditation, listening to music, browsing the internet, cooking, writing, mood chart and journal, hugs, shopping, cinema and telly, blogging and Twitter. I also comfort eat and self harm but, although they do work, I am aware that they are in themselves, self-destructive.

Has your experience with doctors etc been good or bad?

Good all round – occasionally I get frustrated because they just don't understand what I'm trying to say, but that's really down to me. I need to be more articulate.

What's the main thing that changed after you got your diagnosis?

I took a different tack... instead of constantly being on the back foot and living in fear of where my messed up head would take me next, I got proactive and started to learn as much as I could and form strategies to help me maintain my valuable stability. I wasn't as scared of the me inside as I used to be.

Why don't you hide the scars on your arm?

I used to – but then I just decided I was done hiding my mental illness and ergo the self harm. My marks are comparatively small, but if folk do see them and ask I just give them a direct answer. There is never a need to make a big deal out of it. I cover up fresh cuts for a day or so because they may cause distress and I don't want to upset anybody.

Do you find visiting the psychiatrist to be difficult?

I used to. I felt very intimidated. It doesn't bother me now because I go in prepared; I write down relevant info and questions and I bring a pad and pen in case I need to jot anything down. It is so much easier now.

If you are religious, how can you consider suicide?

First off, I would describe myself as spiritual rather than religious, but that's a distinction for another time. The question isn't as simple as it seems but in short, those times when I had been in suicidal crisis I firmly believed that God would understand and forgive me. In the cold light of day the whole philosophical and theological aspects can be examined but not in that dark place; I needed to believe that God would understand, so I made it real.

Do you crack jokes about mental illness?

In close company who know my history, yes – a sense of humour is an important social tool. However, I would be really wary of doing so in a group of strangers – I would hate to be misunderstood, or worse, cause someone offence.

In between episodes are you completely symptom free?

Unfortunately not. Everyone is different, but I continue to have issues such as general anxiety, poor concentration, mild OCD, social anxiety, self-harm, sleep difficulties, poor memory, and distraction... stuff like that.

When you are no longer depressed, do the thoughts of suicide still arise?

Yes – but in my case, usually fleeting. Every day, every single day, even the wonderfully happy ones, the thought creeps in somehow; something you see or hear triggers it. I have become accustomed to it now and find the best way to deal is not to try and ignore it, but to listen to it, acknowledge it and then allow it to pass on. Fighting it only makes it worse. It is what it is. I'm used to that.

Do you think the general public understand what bipolar disorder is?

There is an increasing awareness I think, particularly due to disclosure of some high profile celebrities and some excellent handling of the subject on television; it is however mainly a vague awareness. People seem to understand bipolar by one or two generalisations in the same way that many understand OCD by straightening cans in a food cupboard, diabetes by taking insulin, eating disorders by starving or cancer by losing your hair. It's a start though.

Have you ever had a mixed episode?

Yeah, those can actually be quite distressing – you can get pulled in so many directions, swinging from one extreme to the other many times during just one day and at times there is weird confusion. People around you don't know what's going on or how to react and leave you on your own to deal with it. Thankfully, for me at least, this type of episode is a very rare occurrence.

Do you find peer discussion about bipolar useful?

Yes – incredibly. You can pick up hints on how better to manage your condition and most importantly, you don't feel alone anymore.

Is there anything about TV's portrayal of mental illness that upsets you?

Over all I'd have to say no – they may try to assign too many symptoms to one character sometimes which can give the public a distorted view of an illness. That said, I think it is great that soaps

and films etc are more comfortable approaching the subject; it should ultimately help end stigma. When actual suicides are shown on TV or film, especially those involving cutting, I get very uncomfortable – there's nothing wrong with what they are showing, it's just that it hits a raw nerve and my mind flies off in a direction I don't really want to follow.
My problem; not theirs.

Have you ever deliberately gone against the advice of your key-workers?

Well, I've been asked not to take too much alcohol – that one is actually easy enough – it's the cut down the coffee one that makes me laugh. I survive on coffee in work and I refuse to do without. I'm advised to maintain a regular sleep pattern, but I really don't do so well with that either. The biggie is the meds – there are serious consequences to missing daily meds, but there have been times when I have skipped up to two weeks or more. They call that non-compliance and they really get upset with you when you do it. All I can say is that it made sense at the time.

If you could reclaim one difficult aspect of your bipolar life, what would it be?

Reading – I used to really love reading, but my concentration has been so poor these past few years, I can only manage a few pages at a time. I have my favourite book on my phone now so I still try and dip in when I can.

Do you ever think about how you'll cope when you're much older?

Not in any great detail. I mainly worry about losing Hubby and having to be alone: I joke that if he dies first, I'll kill him.

Do you consider yourself disabled?

Yes – you're considered disabled under the UK Equality Act 2010 and Disability Discrimination Act 2005 (1995) if you have a physical or mental impairment that has a 'substantial' and 'long-term' negative effect on your ability to do normal daily activities. Without going into unnecessary details, I do meet these criteria.
If there's a box on a form I tick it.

Do you believe it's possible to over-think your illness?

A few have tried to tell me that, but I can't allow myself to believe it – I am a bipolar survivor because I choose to think about things, to educate myself and to understand. "To conquer an enemy you must first name him, then with steeled purpose, attack with knowledge of his very soul."

When was the last time you really laughed out loud?

At a Dara O'Briain comedy night in Dublin. The tickets had been a birthday present.

If you've so much trouble concentrating, how are you managing to write this?

It is taking a VERY long time. Months, almost a year. Although I was recently blessed with a period of hypomania. As of typing this, the book is 95% finished. And that, folks, is why I love hypomania.

Do you gamble or drink alcohol in excess?

I am aware that we bipolars are more likely to be drawn to addictive behaviours, but the only gambling I do is a fun lottery or raffle ticket; I do drink, but on the advice of my psychiatrist, have cut right down. In case you're wondering – I don't take recreational drugs either; I have enough trouble dealing with the prescription ones.

What's the most unusual thing you've done lately?

I'm only 45 and I have just finished writing out my wishes regarding my funeral. It is a detailed document giving exact hymns, readings and music for each of the two ceremonies. My tastes are not conventional, so the music files themselves have even been sourced and saved. I did this during a period of hypomania and was not in any way planning my death – just my funeral.

Elaine Fogarty

What's your pet peeve?

Many times over the years, I've been in a situation where I have had cause to be upset, perhaps not greatly so, but upset; I found that my grievances were ignored or played down, because it was assumed that my bipolar mind had misinterpreted the situation or that because of my illness I had over-reacted or indeed imagined the whole thing. Even friends and family who know me really well have done this – unintentionally of course – but they've done it. It has been so hurtful in the past that I of late have decided to keep my mouth shut – just take the hit and ride out situations like these – it's just not worth it. It's a bit like a driver immediately getting blamed for an accident because of an L plate on their window; automatically more culpable because of assumed inexperience and inability. Of course the key word here is 'assumed' and we all know what that is.

Do you find yourself blaming bipolar for all the problems in your life?

When very depressed, that can happen; when stable and thinking more clearly, I'd have to say no. In fact, it's refreshing to have 'normal' problems and stuff to deal with now and then; bizarrely, it can be comforting – reminds me that I'm still part of the human race.

If you could choose one word to describe hypomania, what would it be?

Surreal.

Does your illness scare people?

Yes – It often does. Some will ask questions and talk about it but some just avoid you, sometimes even choosing to talk about you behind your back.

Ever think of writing a book?

Well, thank you... and here it is. They say everyone has a book in them and it just took a gentle nudge from people like you to finally convince me to get mine in print. I believe this unique and very personal approach will help people better understand the bipolar mind and I only hope it reaches the people who need it.

So, what's with the charts and the notes?

Keeping a record of mood shifts and life events helps the professionals provide better treatment; they are so much better informed. It also means patterns can be identified and triggers isolated – with this information plans can be made for how to better cope with the bipolar rollercoaster. It helps me. It helps them.

Knew you were unwell, wanted to text, but didn't know what to say...

That's lovely – it's the contact that's important, not the content, so don't worry. Something simple like – "Thinking of you, hope you feel better soon, I'm here if you need to talk."

Are you an expert on bipolar?

Oh, no – I've simply gathered information and coping strategies over the years that help me cope within my own journey. I'm happy to share what I've learnt but it isn't informed by any professional qualification or scientific study. I don't imply for one minute that my experience is representative of all sufferers; we all have a unique cocktail of symptoms. My story is offered here merely as example.

Do you think a holistic approach to bipolar treatment works?

I know there are many who have successfully used it, experiencing long-term benefits; personally, I prefer just to use elements of it to supplement a more traditional approach.

Do you ever pretend to experience symptoms because it suits a situation?

No – I can't understand why anyone would do that.

Have you ever been tempted to tell key-workers what you thought they wanted to hear?

Well, I hate to admit it, but yes – not only tempted, but I've done it. It's not something I'm proud of.

How do you feel about the use of words like crazy, mad, deranged, demented and insane?

If you begin to look these words up in the dictionary you will be there a while because the definitions just keep pointing you back to one of the others; they are basically the same thing. Mad, for example, is defined as "mentally disturbed, deranged or insane". There is a resurgence of the use of these words and I think it's good that we are reclaiming them. I don't find them derogatory at all and in fact I use some of them myself, for example online – "Welcome to my little blog about mundane minutia and madness".

Is there anything you'd love to do but can't because of your bipolar?

I regret having to give up my yoga teaching, but developments in my condition have meant it is unlikely I'll ever pick it up again. I used to joke that one day I'd go to Amsterdam, head to a little cafe, and get myself huge a slice of cake – guess that's out the window now, too.

Do you trust your own judgements?

When I'm stable I have little reason not to, but just to be on the safe side, I allow myself a cooling off period on major decisions – especially if there is a lot of money involved. Experience with my past behaviour during episodes has taught me to be careful, but it is after all good advice for anyone, with or without a mental illness. I trust those close to me to step in with a 'reality check' if needed and that provides a welcome safety net.

Do the meds actually work?

I can only speak from my perspective, but I'd have to say that, yes – they work. They don't make the mood swings go away completely, after all why would they? Mood swings are normal. I now have the kind of normal mood shifts that everyone has and I also have ones that are bipolar related; the meds usually stop the bipolar swings from moving into the dangerous extremes of old – simply put, they 'take the edge off' I'm very happy with the help my medication has given me. One important issue here – they can only work if you take them.

Do the professionals make things better or worse?

Strange question – I always had the best of support from my key-workers, even when I thought I didn't need it. I appreciate there may be some out there who have had bad experiences, but I've been lucky in regard to those assigned to help me.

Hedgehogging? What on earth is hedgehogging?

When a computer has too many conflicting issues, it freezes and forces shut down and re-boot. I say I'm hedghogging when I feel compelled to do the same, when I need to escape the intensity of my world and find a dark comfy area in which to be alone for a while. Just as a little hedgehog seeks a place in which to hibernate – it's one of my most important coping mechanisms; I usually emerge with clearer perspective and less anxiety.

Do you hear voices?

Not in the sense you mean – I often hear lots of little voices competing for attention inside my head, but they are all me. All different, but all me. I'm aware that that doesn't make sense – welcome to my world.

Is there a pattern to all these episodes?

Everyone is different; I can discern no definite, repeatable pattern to my episodes except for two things – depression and Christmas are best friends and depression follows hypomania like a cart follows a horse.

Are there any perks to having bipolar disorder?

Well, I'm more creative and I do get a postal vote.

You can sometimes go from 0 – hostile in 5 seconds flat. I suppose you're gonna blame that on bipolar disorder as well?

Well, um.... Dare I say ... yes? I can get angry just like anyone else, but because of the bipolar I sometimes jump straight to extremes without even realising it. I'd like to think I don't do it anywhere near as much these days.

What was the last thing to make you cry?

Watching a seal being toyed with and then killed by a whale on TV. I sat on my sofa and pretended the odd tear wasn't rolling down my face; silent sniffs and sobs conspired to keep the secret.

Do you declare your mental illness to prospective employers?

I've been with my current employer 10 years so, since before diagnosis; I've no experience with this. I know disclosing my bipolar disorder to a prospective employer would carry considerable risk and there is still a lot of stigma attached to it; I think though, that I would. I'd take the chance. Besides, if I hoped to be able to ask for reasonable adjustments and ongoing support within the workplace, I'd have to disclose – there is no option.

In conversation, do you find yourself actively looking for ways to be offended?

NO – but I guess I can understand that some folk with my illness can become hypersensitive, and vehemently defend their bipolar identity against even perceived stigma. I guess if you're prepared for a fight, every noise is going to sound like a starting bell.

What jobs have you done – paid or unpaid?

Sales assistant in a shoe store – Sales assistant in a jewellery store – Assistant manager in a jewellery store – Receptionist with the housing executive – Telephonist with the housing executive – Cub scout leader – Venture scout leader – Brownie leader – Admin assistant with the housing executive – Repairs clerk – Trainee housing assessment officer with the housing executive – Training officer in a jeweller's store – Children's summer camp supervisor – Volunteer in a club for the blind and partially sighted – Teacher of art and crafts – Manager in a jewellery store – Volunteer in a charity shop – Youth club leader – Yoga teacher – Sunday school teacher – Relaxation Therapist – CD production and sales – Line worker in a food factory – Door to door catalogue sales – Raynet volunteer – Child minder – Market stall seller – Children's evangelist – Personal yoga instructor – Machine operator in a food factory – Sales assistant in a bookstore – Fundraising volunteer with a cancer charity – Sales assistant in a different jewellery store – Sales assistant in a corner shop – Home visit volunteer – Line worker in a large scale bakery – Senior sales assistant in a furniture/fancy goods store – Volunteer in a different charity shop – Santa's elf – Receptionist in a furniture wholesalers – Admin assistant in a furniture wholesalers – Volunteer in yet another charity shop – Author.

Is there a link between sleep patterns and bipolar episodes?

I'm no expert but here's what I know: sleep deprivation can cause me to shift into hypomania & hypomania causes my need for sleep to evaporate. There's nothing for it but to try and maintain a regular sleep pattern.

Have you ever taken part in any studies?

No – just small surveys as they as they come my way. Sometimes though, the answers are more confusing than the questions.

Are you naturally a creature of habit or do you deliberately seek routine because of the bipolar disorder?

I've found that pinning my day to a proved routine is immensely helpful in easing my general bipolar symptoms, as well as the anxiety and the OCD. The best way I can describe it is, that it feels like being able to dim the lights in a harshly lit room.

What do you mean, 'you've got it all worked out'?

It's hard to explain – sometimes I feel like I can see everything around me oh so clearly, can solve all the problems. It all makes sense. I get upset with people who don't understand me. It doesn't happen often and it's most likely the hypomania talking but at the time it is totally real.

Can you still give blood whilst taking all those meds?

Yes. That is, I believe so. I was told not so long ago by my service that, providing you are on a 'maintenance treatment' and are well on the day of donation, then all should be OK. It isn't guaranteed though because the session officer can, on assessment, decline. They told me that the same would apply for marrow harvesting.

Do you ever feel sorry for yourself?

Yes – there's no point in lying about it – I do. Sometimes it all gets a little too hard to live with and I begin to look around, convincing myself that everyone else has it much better, and that life is deliberately picking on me. It's getting easier to challenge thoughts like these since I was introduced to cognitive behavioural therapy.

How long have you been in your current relationship?

I've been with Colin 28½ years – we've been married for 21 of those and we still hold hands! He's the rock that I cling to.

Have you ever been told to 'pull yourself together'?

Yes – it hurts – but it isn't usually born of malice; there are a lot of people out there who have no understanding of mental illness. I used to get angry but now I stay calm.

Sometimes you're really quiet. Sometimes you never shut up. What's with that?

It's the moods, and sorry, I don't always realise I'm doing it. Everyone does this to some degree, but when you notice me do it in extreme, then it's most likely the bipolar causing it. When I retreat into myself like that it most likely means that I'm depressed: when I'm overly jittery and chatty it most likely means I'm hypomanic.

Will you be taking those pills for the rest of your life?'

Possibly – but I'd much rather do that than live life the way it used to be.

Do you hallucinate?

No. Thankfully, that is one symptom I've never experienced. I've heard it can be quite distressing.

What was the biggest change in your relationship when you started treatment?

Hubby and I don't really argue much anymore – I don't miss those really intense times. Looking back, I can totally see how the big spoon of bipolar was stirring the pot.

Was the psych ward like it is on TV?

I suppose it depends on what TV you've seen. If you mean padded cells, barred windows and tyrannical staff, then – no, my ward was nothing like that. I felt quite safe and comfortable there and the staff were generally very nice. I wasn't on an intensive care ward.

Why do you not watch the news anymore?

It usually makes me upset. I'm hypersensitive and hyperemotional; even though it's just a newscast, it can be quite intense for me. Other people think I'm a bid odd because of this, but I'm just removing myself from a difficult situation.

What do you think about Marvin?

The Hitchhikers Guide to the Galaxy is actually my favourite book and, up until it was explained to me, I believed that Marvin was exactly what all manically depressed people were – dreary, miserable and constantly moaning. I fell for the stereotype. He doesn't upset me now that I know the truth of the condition – in fact it rather makes me laugh. I've had to develop a sense of humour about my illness – it sometimes helps when nothing else does.

How did your very first appointment go?

I was scared and intimidated; I wouldn't even go in alone. I don't remember much except that he asked me who the current prime minister was and I genuinely couldn't tell him. Ouch!

Do they use ECT to treat bipolar?

ECT is a treatment that uses electrical current to influence brain function. Although much maligned, it has proven extremely beneficial for some, relieving symptoms of mania, severe depression and suicidal risk. I have never had ECT treatment.

How do you handle panic attacks?

Stupid as it sounds, the best thing to do is try not to actually have them. I often adjust my plans to avoid situations known to give me trouble. If it's too late and I find myself in the middle of a panic attack, then I call on my breathing techniques – slowing the breathing usually slows everything else down too. If the calm breathing just isn't doing its job, then I reach for the medication I carry with me wherever I go. I hate panic attacks – knowing that everyone is staring makes it so much worse.

What, if any philosophical question has you bipolar condition lead you to consider?

Well, quite obviously, the duality of existence and the quest for balance. I've also put in many a long night considering the nature of identity and indeed, perception and its role in creating reality. I still haven't quite decided whether or not I truly believe in fate and my spiritual self is still struggling to know God better.

Has your condition made you more empathetic?

I'd say so, Yes.

Do you have any difficulty coping with day to day stuff?

Well, the list here could be quite long, but as an example – I don't do well alone. I can't just jump in the car and go where ever I like – I can't just walk into a strange bar or restaurant – I can't take public transport on my own – I can't easily attend appointments in unfamiliar places – I need someone with me. Although, at a push, I can do some of these things on my own, given the choice, I'd always have someone with me. I'm 45 and it's quite embarrassing to admit this, but none the less, it's true.

Do you think older generations have difficulty dealing with mental illness?

Not so much a difficulty dealing with it – but rather – talking about it. In my grandparents' time I'd have been labelled as 'bad with my nerves' and with that generalisation, it would never have been talked about again. In my parents' time it would have been referred to occasionally, but rarely discussed at length. People of my own generation and indeed younger, are beginning to combat stigma and be more accepting of folk with mental illness; it is the beginning of a long journey.

Do you ever wish you'd never been open about your bipolar?

Every now and then something happens that makes me feel as if I'm under a huge spotlight – it's difficult to adequately describe how uncomfortable that can be. Overall though, I'd have to say no. I'm glad I found the courage to be open about my mental illness and I'm very happy to escape the suffocating influence of secrecy.

What's the worst thing anyone has ever said to you?

"Oh, for God's sake, just do it and stop moaning about it."

Have you ever used any of the telephone support lines?

Yes – with varying degrees of success. For the most part my experience has been very good and those crisis help lines have actually saved my life more than once. We need to remember though, that the voice on the other end is a flesh and blood human, and as such, can have a bad day themselves – a couple of times I have hung up from one of those calls feeling worse than when I dialled in. I wish it weren't true but it is. Would I still recommend them? YES, Yes and yes. They do a difficult yet crucial job very well; they listen when no one else will.

If you could choose one word to describe depression, what would it be?

Suffocating.

Any hints for other bipolar sufferers?

Never leave the house without your emergency numbers. Throw the scales out; if you obsess it only gets worse. Write, sing, draw, paint... anything, just find a way to vent. Give yourself a cooling off period with all major decisions. Take the meds, no, really, TAKE the meds. Be honest. Stop trying to be normal; there's no such thing!

Are you ever embarrassed by your mental illness?

I try not to, but sometimes I do feel that way.

Have you ever found yourself saying or doing anything inappropriate?

Yes – I often engage my mouth before my brain has had time to kick in. For example, when watching a suicide scene on television with friends, announcing loudly "Well, she's doing that wrong. She should.............."

What's the most helpful thing anyone has ever said to you?

"You know girl, I wouldn't want you any other way." {Arms outstretched for a hug.}

How do you tell a normal mood swing from a bipolar one?

Well, that can be difficult because they sort of feel the same at first. A bipolar mood shift is simply one that becomes more intense or lasts significantly longer than a normal one. There it is again – that word normal – I hate it. However, I know I have to recognise the 'normalcy' in my life and not be tempted to assign meaning to every little mood. Not all bad days are because of the bipolar – I'm getting better at telling the difference.

How do you deal with the weight gain?

To be honest, I don't deal that well at all. I have trouble losing weight and it drains my self-esteem. At the moment I am attending a 'Slimming World' group and because of that support, I'm actually making progress. It's like any other challenge – peer support is essential if you are going to succeed.

I've heard bipolar can make you reckless with money – is that true?

It is a common indicator for mania/hypomania but not everyone actually experiences it. I am troubled with this but have gradually become better at minimising risk; I allow myself a cooling off period on all major purchases and work from lists where possible when shopping. For me, the 'damage' within one episode is usually quite manageable but I remember, during one three week episode a few years ago, spending more than 5 times my weekly wage on unnecessary or ill-timed purchases.

Do you object to people using the term bipolar simply to describe a person who has difficulty making up their mind – Yes, No, Maybe sort of thing?

No – it's usually pretty obvious that no harm is intended – besides – it often quite funny. I try not to take myself too seriously.

Do you have a specific suicide plan?

There no point in lying. Yes – once a plan is made it cannot be unmade. It is extremely important to point out thought, that HAVING a plan is not the same as USING a plan. It is a truth that is not easily explained.

Have your untreated symptoms become better or worse over time?

Over 30 years, I'd definitely have to say worse, but it wasn't a comfortable linear progression. If I were to plot a graph, it would show random spikes leading to a plateau that then becomes the new baseline for an extended period. These spikes all seem to occur around the time of a major life event or a spontaneous breakdown.

Can children have bipolar disorder?

I'm unable to fully answer. This is such a controversial issue that even the professionals disagree; the problem is, many of the noted 'symptoms' can, in the eyes of others, be attributed to the expected irrational and intense behaviours of a normal growing child. The last I heard, America led the way in diagnosis of young children (prescribing anti-psychotics and other mood stabilising drugs to children as young as four) but it is certainly not the only country to do so.

At diagnosis, how did you deal with the massive influx of information about bipolar disorder?

I was very overwhelmed. The basics were well explained but I was also advised to go online and visit the sites listed on the little leaflets I'd been given: I was told to take my time and let it sink in a bit and then ask as many questions as necessary. While still a little dazed, I began to do just that. This approach worked well for me and I have continued to learn this way.

Do you experience poor memory?

The short answer is yes. But there's a but – it's not actually a poor memory issue in the purest sense. To put it as simply as I can, I don't remember things well because my distracted or uninterested state means my subconscious isn't really paying attention! Simple as that... I spend a lot of time just skimming over life and sadly many of the details just don't sink in. A good example of this is facial recall in combination with name recall – everyone experiences this problem now and then, but I struggle every single time. I could be in a car on a Monday and not be able to give you make or colour on a Tuesday. Listening to the news upsets me so I rarely do it, but on those rarest of occasions, I find my recall is vague. The simple 'day to day' solution to the little memory inconveniences is to carry a note pad and of course my OCD self just loves lists!

Has your employer made 'reasonable adjustments' to help you?

Yes. When my diagnosis came to light, they immediately offered support; after discussion, minor but welcome changes were made to my job description. I have an 'open door 'invitation to discuss any difficulties that may arise and I check in regularly with one particular person. Time off needed for appointments etc is understood and supported, and they have assisted me in finding ways to combat stress or moments of overwhelm during episodes. I am fully aware that this kind of support is still rare in the workplace and it is always greatly appreciated.

Have you seen the film *One Flew Over the Cuckoo's Nest*? Is it really like that?

I can't speak to other's experience in mental health treatment, but my own was absolutely nothing like that. Good film though. Jack was brilliant.

What emergency numbers do you carry?

I'm always afraid of finding myself without them, so I don't carry a note in my bag, I have them printed on a handkerchief that I tuck into my clothing. My numbers are –
Home …Mobile…Husband mobile…Husband work…Parents home…Mum's mobile…Dad's mobile…Sister mobile… Sister home… Sister work…Colin's parents home… Colin's parents mobile…Best mate mobile…GP surgery…Out of hours doctor…Community mental health team…Police non-emergency number…Samaritans…2 taxi numbers.
It also carries my address, diagnosis and a lithium notification

Do your episodes appear in conjunction with the changing seasons?

As a rule, no, not really – however, as with the rest of the population, winter can be more challenging. The Christmas and New Year festivities are difficult for me, not only because of the social anxiety, but because I feel suffocated by other people's happiness; it stirs up a lot of issues. Generally, I'd say three out of every five Christmas seasons are spent in a deep depressive episode.

Ok, so we've established you're a social media fan, but is it helpful in dealing with the bipolar?

Overall, I'd have to say the peer support is invaluable. There is one thing though that I don't like. Sadly, some accounts choose to place a photograph of their self harm AS THEIR PROFILE PIC or AVATAR. I just don't have the words to express how inappropriate and dangerous this is. Embedded links are there to be used; I don't understand what the motive for this behaviour might be.

What exactly are they testing for when you give a sample every three months?

The main thing is lithium level, but in my experience they also test liver function and thyroid function. I've also had hormone profile and cholesterol checked.

How do you know those folk online are really in crisis and not just attention seeking?

Well, truthfully, you can never know for sure. I'd much rather assume their post is genuine and offer what assistance I can – rather a waste of time than a waste of life.

Are there still some conversations you'd rather not have?

Well, yes. There are some people in my life who struggle to understand my mental illness, or more accurately, the suicidal ideation and self harm. Although I'm more than happy to talk, I am very conscious that they would feel uncomfortable hearing it; I respect that and only discuss my bipolar experiences when they raise the issue themselves.

Do your key-workers always agree regarding treatment?

I can't answer that. It's highly unlikely they'd ever tell me directly if there was some kind of disagreement regarding correct treatment; it would be extremely unprofessional to do so. My observations to date lead me to believe that they communicate well and do work together to offer me the most suitable treatment.

Does it annoy you to answer the same questions time and time again?

No – questions show people are taking a genuine interest in either me personally or mental illness in general. That can only be a good thing and I am happy to do my bit to combat stigma through education and empathy.

When you come across the **TRIGGER** tag on social network posts, what do you do?

I trust the judgement of the author, and if I'm feeling delicate or at risk, I do as intended – I skip on by – I don't read it. When I am more stable, I will however, read on because I'm always interested in how other people deal with their demons. It took me about a year to develop this strength – when new to MH forums etc, curiosity usually wins out.

Are you sure that bipolar is the right diagnosis for you?

When they began to explain the intricacies of it, all the fear and confusion of my life just slotted into place. Bipolar II perfectly explains the difficulties I live with and I'm confident that it is indeed the correct diagnosis. I don't need to stretch or invent things to fit my diagnosis – it makes sense just the way it is.

Having been caught out by the sneaky question during assessment once before, can you tell me now who is the current UK Prime minister?

Oh, right, very funny... 6 years on and we're not going to let that one go are we? It's.. It's... I can picture his face... The other guy too... What is his name?
No... Damn...That's so embarrassing. I guess there are some things that really will never change.

Are you able to manage your meds ok?

How well I manage depends on how well I am feeling; unfortunately right when I need them most, I often find myself being erratic in my taking of them. I know how serious it can be to mess with the meds routine but I do have difficulties none the less. I can genuinely forget. I can get confused. I can deliberately stop, even deliberately change dosages. Most of the time though, I try hard to do things right. When very unwell, I once had the huge pre-prepared blister packs direct from the chemist all sorted and ready. That was helpful up to a point. Mostly now I stay on top of things by using one of those little cases with a divided box for each day. I also have some benzos for use as needed.

Do you regret leaving the retail management sector?

No – I enjoyed it, I was good at it, but I needed to back away from the stress. I had to put my health first.

Is it true that you bipolars are wired to be more promiscuous?

Lack of inhibition and hyper-sexuality can occur in mania (or hypomania) This, combined with lapses in judgement can invite promiscuity but it is by no means a blanket symptom; some never experience it. I have had to work hard to manage my hypomania symptoms and minimise risk.

Do you cry easily?

I used to cry easily, deeply and often. I complain regularly now that the meds have stolen my tears. I find myself needing to cry, craving the cleansing and healing influence of tears yet almost always unable to do it. This is a constant irritation to me.

Have you ever used your mental illness as a weapon?

No – No matter how much someone upset me, I would never try to 'guilt' them into submission. I would suffer more from that action than they would, for I would have to become the worst version of myself to do it.

What's the best lie you've ever told to get out of a psych assessment/admission/similar?

Sure, yeah, feeling a lot better, the dreams have stopped and well, I'm still low but at least I don't feel like killing myself.

Do you not think you're a bit old for all this cr*p?

I'm 45 but the bipolar doesn't care; it's been with me since I was a teen and I'm quite sure it is planning on hanging around. My illness isn't something I can outgrow. It really isn't about age - I speak to teens online as peers; we have a shared experience and shared challenges.

What do you think about the way TV cop shows often have bipolar suspects for murder and assault?

I would have to say part of me is a little concerned that the general public will form hasty assumptions about our illness, but then I have to be realistic. Any shows I have seen have based it on a presentation of actual bipolar symptoms and usually stating that the suspect had not been taking their meds. It is plausible - regrettable - but plausible. Fair representation of mental ill-health must by definition include the downside. This happens with other conditions too.

Have you ever photographed your areas of self harm?

Yes - Not habitually, but I do have some photos (Some are more graphic than others.) I'm not sure why I keep them. I simply feel that I may need them some day.

Do you feel lonely?

I feel lonely in a crowded life when my mood dips I am nostalgic for my younger days. My social circle is so small now it is almost a straight line but I can just about live with that. There are those who are truly close to me and that is enough.

Totally open you say... Has there ever been a question you refused to answer?

I will not answer a question that relates to specific details of any suicidal crisis or indeed, of my plans themselves. I can't share them because that would render my plans useless. It would also be unfair to risk triggering someone else who may be struggling.

Is there any event in your past that has left you scarred?

I had a gun held to my head once during a robbery. I won't be forgetting that feeling anyway soon - I still have the occasional frightening dream.

You do realise that your decision to be totally open about your mental illness means EVERYONE will read EVERTHING; It will be out there FOR THE REST OF YOUR LIFE. Family, neighbours, employers, friends and colleagues, health workers etc etc -
Are you ready for that?

It is a risk. I understand that, but I am just so done playing things down and hiding. The stigma of mental illness will only end if people are prepared to take that risk. I have nothing to be ashamed of and I am ready to start talking.

How long after your last suicidal crisis were you back at work and trying to function?

On the morning of the 3rd day - It was really difficult and yet it was like nothing had happened. It was really weird. Truthfully, I didn't get much done that day for I was terribly distracted by thoughts of how close I had come. I was pretty delicate for the week or so afterwards but an opportunity never really arose to discuss it so I struggled on alone.

Do you think pets have a positive influence on a mentally ill person?

Yes, they have an incredibly positive influence on anyone willing to engage with them, not just the mentally ill. Cats and dogs in particular are consistently reported as sensing 'a bad patch' and initiating contact so they can comfort their owner. It has been noted that this often happens before surrounding humans have even picked up that there is a problem. The unconditional love a pet offers is wonderful and I know in my own experience there were dark and despairing days I would never have made it out of bed but for the hungry protestations of my cat.

When was the last time you had an anxiety attack?

About ten days ago.

When was the last time you thought about your suicide plan?

Yesterday.

When was the last time someone engaged you in conversation about mental health?

About four days ago.

When was the last time you cried yourself to sleep?

About a week ago.

When was the last time someone said something derogatory, cruel or hurtful to you about your mental illness?

About a month ago.

When was the last time you self harmed?

Last night.

When was the last time you felt scared/overwhelmed by your mental state?

About three days ago.

What are the statistics for mental illness?

The generally accepted UK statistic is that 1 in 4 people, yes, 1 in 4, will have some kind of mental ill-health issue in any given year. This figure is fluid and sadly is heading closer to 1 in 3.

Do you think everyone should be open about their mental illness?

I think everyone should at least consider it, but stigma is deeply ingrained in our society still, and I can understand why many feel more comfortable not sharing. A mental ill-health diagnosis can be scary and confusing and we must all deal the best way we know how. I will not judge another's choice.

Can you make sense of any of those acronyms and abbreviations?

I've become used to reading and using them. Below, I've brought together all I can remember seeing these past few years as I navigated various reading materials, forums and social network sites world-wide; not all are in current use by professionals; some are simply born of convenience when chatting online with like-minded folk. There will of course be omissions – for that I'm sorry.

Mental health related acronyms and abbreviations

A	Admittance
A&E	Accident and emergency
AB	Anti-biotic
AD	Advance directive
AD	Anti-depressant
AD	Anxiety disorder
ADD	Attention deficit disorder
ADHD	Attention deficit-hyperactivity disorder
ADL	Activities of daily living
ADR	Adverse drug reaction
AE	As expected
ALF	Acute liver failure
AMHD	Advance mental health directive
AN	Anorexia Nervosa
AP	Active participation
AP	Anti-psychotic
APPT	Appointment
AR	Adverse reaction
AS	Attempted suicide
ASL	Active social life
ATC	Around the clock
BAD	Bipolar affective disorder
BDZ	Benzodiazepine
BL	Body language
BP	Bipolar disorder
BPD	Borderline personality disorder
BT	Blood test
BZ	Benzodiazepine
BZD	Benzodiazepine
CAN	Child abuse and neglect
CAT	Cognitive analytic therapy
CBT	Cognitive behavioural therapy
CFH	Cry for help
CHL	Crisis helpline
CMHT	Community mental health team
COBPD	Childhood onset bipolar disorder
CP	Care plan
CPN	Community psychiatric nurse
CR	Constructed reality
CRHT	Crisis resolution home treatment

CS	Coping strategy
D(EL)	Delusions/Delusional
DBT	Dialectical behavioural therapy
DC	Discharge
DDA	Disability discrimination act (2005) (1995)
DLA	Disability living allowance
DNA	Did not attend
DSH	Deliberate self harm
DV	Domestic violence
DX	Diagnosis
EA	Equality act (2010)
ECT	Electroconvulsive therapy
ED	Eating disorder
EDNOS	Eating disorder (not otherwise specified)
EEG	Electroencephalogram
EI	Early intervention
EI	Emotional intelligence
EMW	Early morning waking
EP	Episode
ESA	Employment and Support Allowance
FMH	Family medical history
FMHH	Family mental health history
FS	Family situation
GAD	Generalized anxiety disorder
GI	Good insight
GP	General Practitioner (The family doctor)
H(AL)	Hallucinations
HA	Hospital admittance
HAT	Holistically augmented therapy
HCP	Health care provider
HCP	Home care plan
HFF	Hope for the future
HI	Homicidal ideation
HL	Home life
HS	Home situation
HSE	Health service executive (Ireland)
HV	Home visit
ICAS	Independent complaints & advocacy service
IP	In patient
KW	Key-worker
LOC	Loss of concentration
LOI	Lack of insight
LOL	Loss of libido

LTC	Long term condition
LTT	Long term treatment
MAU	Medical admissions unit
MD	Manic depression
MD	Mood disorder
MDD	Manic depressive disorder
MEDS	Medication
MH	Mental health
MHA	Mental health assessment
MHH	Mental health history
MHST	Mental health support team
MHSU	Mental health service user
MHT	Mental health trust
MI	Mental illness
MPD	Multiple personality disorder
MRN	Medication review needed
MS	Mood stabiliser
NA	Next appointment
NAMI	National alliance on mental illness (US)
NC	No change
NC	Non communicative
NC	Non compliance
NC	Non co-operative
NEC	Not elsewhere classified
NF	Not forthcoming
NHS	National health service (UK)
NHSD	National health service direct
NO	Negative outlook
NOK	Next of kin
NOS	Not otherwise specified
NR	Non-responsive
OBS	Observation
OCD	Obsessive compulsive disorder
OD	Overdose
ODAAT	One day at a time
OG	On going
OOH	Out of hours
OP	Out patient
OT	Occupational therapist (therapy)
P(A)	Paranoia
PALS	Patient advice and liaison service
PBO	Placebo
PC	Poor concentration
PD	Panic disorder

PD	Personality disorder
PDOC	Psychiatrist
PEC	Pre-existing condition
PH	Previous history
PICU	Psychiatric intensive care unit
PIP	Personal Independence Payment
PN	Psychiatric nurse
PO	Positive outlook
POM	Peace of mind
PS	Peer support
PSYC(H)	Psychiatrist
PSYC(H)	Psychologist
PTSD	Post traumatic stress disorder
R(EL)	Relapse
RA	Risk assessment
RLS	Restless leg syndrome
RNR	Rest and relaxation
RTT	Referral to treatment
RV	Review
S(UI)	Service user involvement
SA	Social anxiety
SA	Substance abuse
SA	Suicide attempt
SAD	Seasonal affective disorder
SAD	Social anxiety disorder
SAR	Serious adverse reaction
SCAD	Schizoaffective disorder
SCZ	Schizophrenia
SD	Sleep disruption
SDX	Self diagnosis
SE	Self esteem
SE	Side effect
SI	Self injury
SI	Suicidal ideation
SIP	Support in place
SITREP	Situation report
SM	Stress management
SN	Social networking
SNRI	A type of anti-depressant
SP	Sleep pattern
SP	Social phobia
SPMI	Severe and persistent mental illness
SR	Suicide risk
SS	School situation

SSRI	A common type of anti-depressant
SU	Service user
SUI	Suicide
SW	Suicide watch
SY(M)	Symptoms
SZ	Schizophrenia
TAU	Treatment as usual
TDOC	Therapist/Counsellor/Psychologist
TE	Therapeutic effect
TL	Therapeutic level
TT	Talking therapy
TX	Treatment/therapy
VA	Voluntary admittance
WG	Weight gain
WL	Weight loss
WS	Work situation

Medication dosage & directions

Examples only -
Exact acronyms/abbreviations can vary from doctor to doctor.

AC	Before meals
AD	Up to
AM	Morning
BD	Twice daily
BID	Twice a day
CC	With food
EMP	As directed
EOD	Every other day
HS	At bedtime
NOCT	Night
PC	After meals
PM	Evening /night
PRN	As required
Q4H	Every four hours
QAM	Every morning
QD	Once a day
QHS	Every night at bedtime
QN	Every night
QOD	Every other day
TID	Three times a day
OTC	Over the counter
POM	Prescription only medicine

There is an instinctual language to colour. These are the colours used in the earlier journal entry along with the emotional state attributed.

Red = Passion, Excitement
Crimson = Anger, Irritability
Yellow = Happiness, laughter
Orange = Hypomania
Black = Suicidal
Grey = Depression
Green = Mellow, Content
Brown = Fear, Anxiety
Blue = Sadness
Purple = Frustration, Confusion
Pink = Love Cream = Invisibility
Peach = Conformity
White = Hope
Gold = Success, Stability, Achievement
Silver = Imagination
Lemon = Plans, Dreams
Rose = Hugs, Kisses, Intimacy
Navy = Responsibility, commitment

If you are a fan of the television program *Inside the actor's studio* you will remember the questions that James Lipton always asked. Of course the idea is originally that of Bernard Pivot. Since I'm in a sharing mood, I thought it would be rather fun to take a crack at it myself.

What is your favourite word?
Hope

What is your least favourite word?
Disconnected

What turns you on (creatively, spiritually or emotionally)?
Hugs

What turns you off?
Lies

What is your favourite curse word?
B*ll*cks

What sound or noise do you love?
Heavy rain

What sound or noise do you hate?
Two pieces of polystyrene rubbing together

What profession other than your own would you like to attempt?
Occupational therapist

What profession would you not like to do?
Chef

If Heaven exists, what would you like to hear God say when you arrive at the Pearly Gates?
Come on in, I can explain it all.

~ ~ ~ ~ ~

And so ends my little book about mundane minutia and madness; it's been nice connecting like this, but if you want to chat some more you can contact me.

bipolarlainey@hotmail.co.uk
Follow @bipolarlainey
Also - Check out the dedicated site
www.diaryofabipolarsurvivor.com
Or my blog   bipolarlainey.blog.co.uk

bipdarlainey . wordpress. com

Find me on facebook and perhaps even join our Private Mental Health Related Group on site
www.facebook.com/bipolarlainey

"Dear God of many names,
Protect your children tonight wherever they are sleeping.
Let them know that the world does not have to be like this.
Place a kiss upon each of their foreheads
And remind them oh so gently
That there are reasons to be hopeful
And reasons for them to dream beautiful dreams."

(Author unknown)

Elaine Fogarty

Lightning Source UK Ltd.
Milton Keynes UK
UKOW041249200613

212572UK00001B/2/P